Chronic Asthma & Me

Chronic Asthma & Me

Emilia Fusco

iUniverse, Inc.
New York Lincoln Shanghai

Chronic Asthma & Me

iUniverse books may be ordered through booksellers or by contacting:

iUniverse
2021 Pine Lake Road, Suite 100
Lincoln, NE 68512
www.iuniverse.com
1-800-Authors (1-800-288-4677)

ISBN-13: 978-0-595-36854-9 (pbk)
ISBN-13: 978-0-595-81266-0 (ebk)
ISBN-10: 0-595-36854-9 (pbk)
ISBN-10: 0-595-81266-X (ebk)

Printed in the United States of America

My Nonna Theresa Salerno

My grandmother was the epitome of a strong woman. I could never do justice in writing about her many wonderful qualities, because she was such an amazing woman. She truly was a "Grand" mother. When you were in her presence, you felt reassured that everything would be okay. She had a special warmth about her that reminded a person of home. She always enjoyed a good laugh or a good movie. But more than anything, she enjoyed being around her children and grandchildren. She was most proud of her family. That sense of love and pride was a value she always stressed to each and every one of us.

As a child, my grandmother grew up without a mother, but had a strong bond with her father and her three brothers. She lost one brother at an early age to a high fever, but always kept the memory of him in her heart. I can recall conversations with her in which the recollection of her lost brother brought tears of sadness to her eyes.

She married my grandfather in 1949, and together they decided to emigrate to the United States. They started a life together in Brooklyn, New York, and were blessed with three wonderful children. Little did they know the trials and tribulations they would have to overcome, living in a foreign country, with the usual struggles of everyday life made more difficult because of the language barrier. Regardless, they worked and raised their family day by day.

At the age of 42, my grandmother developed bronchial asthma. She traveled several times a week to different doctors and pulmonary specialists. She struggled daily with asthma, and such simple things as laughing, walking, and climbing a few steps became difficult. She was immediately put on heavy doses of cortisone, a drug with several negative side effects, such as thinning of the bones and weight gain. She was prescribed Albuterol, Theo-Dour, many doses of antibiotics, and she slept with a nebulizer next to her bed. She had difficulty sleeping in bed due to her severe asthma. Her sleeping difficulties escalated to the point that she had to buy an electric bed similar to a hospital bed so that she could elevate her head at night. Because we were a very tight-knit family we experienced her suffering first-hand on a daily basis. All the grandchildren lived with the fear that we would lose our grandmother. As the years went by, my grandmother's asthma became increasingly problematic. My family and I can recall many, many trips to hospitals and doctor's offices in an effort to ease her pain and her struggle with asthma. It bothered her to know that her family was worried about her. If you met my grandmother, you would know you had met an angel, because she was the most selfless person in the world. She never wanted the focus to be on her, but rather wished to have the spotlight on her children and grandchildren. She did things for others without a second thought—she would cook feasts to feed an army, her neighbors, the elderly, and children. She would buy gifts without a reason, sneak money in the palm of your hand and walk a step behind with a smile on her face so everyone would be happy. But her step behind was due to her asthma.

Nonna, we love you and we miss you so much!!
Your granddaughter, Sandra Ferreri.

My Mother Theresa Salerno

My mother was close to death more than once with this terrible disease. She suffered so much she would try anything to get relief from her constant agony. Once she traveled to the far away city of Livorno for treatment by a specialist. Although it was unusual for a woman to travel alone, because she was a brave woman, my mother went and tried the procedure. The procedure was done while my mother was awake and far away from her family.

For a few months then she was able to walk and laugh, although she continued to suffer with her asthma. In order to for the treatments that were performed in Italy to continue to be of benefit, my mother needed to return to Italy every six months for additional treatment. This need to be away from her family for an extended period of time was a great hardship, because her priority was to feed and care for her children. Therefore, she sacrificed her health by staying where she was needed, and she continued to live with the terrible disease. We could only watch helplessly as our mother, grandmother, and friend, a woman with so much strength, become weakened by such a terrible, yet common disease.

There came a time in her life where she could barely walk from one room to another without losing her breath. There came a time where doing puzzles helped to distract her and ease her pain in the middle of the night, a time when only the promise of an upcoming family gathering gave her the will to survive. She feared dying from asthma. And yet, that's exactly what happened. And there was nothing anyone could do to help. She would only ask that someone help until she looked into the eyes of God and could just breathe.

Asthma is terrible illness that takes the life of so many and makes a very ordinary day unbearable to live. If there is one wish my family and I have, it is that no one should ever have to watch a loved one suffer on a daily basis the way we watched our beloved mother, grandmother and friend suffer.

Ma, we love you and we miss you so much!!
Love, your daughter, Katy.

My Cousin Theresa Salerno

As I write my cousin's story about her experiences with asthma, I remember when she and I spoke on the phone about our experiences with asthma and how difficult our lives were. My cousin Theresa lived in New York, and I lived in Boston, but whenever we could, we would visit each other. Earlier in our lives, my asthma was somewhat less serious than hers, but as the years went by, when we visited each other, the chorus of our wheezing was like a symphony of suffering. It broke my heart to hear her wheezing on the phone. I miss her phone calls and her loving friendship in my life.

We met a few months after I came to this country. She was my first cousin's wife, and yet we came to care and love each other like two sisters and best friends. When her asthma became more serious, the only thing she was concerned and worried about was that she wanted to see her children married before something happened to her. Well, God granted her wish. She lived long enough to see all three children happily married, and even helped her children raise their children.

My dear cousin, my dear friend! Your long and hard road struggling with asthma is finished; now you are at peace with God and your loved ones. No more struggles with your asthma, no more wheezing, no more suffering. I never got a chance to say goodbye to you, and I am filled with regret now! I want you to know you are always going to be in my heart.

With love, your cousin Emilia Fusco.

ACKNOWLEDGEMENTS

To my husband, Peter, for his love and support in my time of need. I feel so guilty for being so sick all those years. I want you to know your love and the love from our children has helped me to be where I am today. Today my Asthma is much more in control and I feel so blessed to have you by my side and in my life. God keep you safe.

To my son, Alberto for being such a big man in his teenage years. Thank you for spending so much time with me in the hospital emergency room and for loving me no matter what. You came with me to the hospital at age 17 to see Dr. Fanta. He introduced you to a physical therapist to learn about Chest PT. How very proud you made me and what a good job you did. To my daughter in-law Kristine, for how good you are to me. Thank you to both of you for giving us two beautiful granddaughters, Cara Mia & Gianna Maria.

To my daughter Silvia for being so understanding. At age 14 you had to deal with a lot. I spent so much time away from you being in the hospital with my Asthma. Every time I left home in the ambulance, the only thing keeping me strong was you and your brother's eyes. They were always scared for me and full of tears. I knew I needed to get better. You are the best daughter and friend any mother could hope to have. Thank you to my son-in-law, Shawn, for always being willing to take me to the hospital. Thank you to both of you for giving us a beautiful grandson, Anthony Michael.

To Dr. Christopher Fanta, I want to thank you for being my doctor for so many years. The day I came to your office for the first time on July 21, 1988, that was my lucky day. You have been my doctor, my asthma teacher and most of all, my friend. You have given me so much acknowledgement and care for my asthma. Thank you for providing me with information to write this book. I feel so blessed to know a teacher like you.

Finally, I want to thank you God for having blessed me with the love and care from my family. Thank you God for giving me such an excellent doctor, Dr. Christopher Fanta, for without his care and dedication I never would have made it through.

Thank you,

Emilia Fusco

<u>My name is Emilia Fusco. I have chronic ASTHMA</u>

I was born and raised in Italy, in the small town of Montepaone, with a population of 4,406, in the province of Catanzaro. Its territory rises from the sea to an altitude of about 367 meters and covers an area close to 17 km from Montepaone Lido. The beach is 3.5 km and the town is 32 km from Catanzaro Provincia. Our costumes are colorful and very traditional.

Calabria is the southern most region of Italy, the ankle and toe of the "boot"—a rugged peninsula where grapevines, fig, and olive trees cling to the arid mountainsides, and where the memorable sea crash against the cliffs and coastline, with long, and intricate west all at once. Calabria is one of the most astonishingly beautiful parts of the world.

For a millennium, the people here have made pottery, spun wool, knitted, and laced garments. They've milked their goats, made fresh cheese, bread, rolled pasta, and fermented wine and oil. The people of Calabria also made beautiful handicrafts, artwork, wood work, ceramic, gold jewels, stone, copper and wrought iron. There is also a fabric made with beautiful designs and embroidery.

<u>Let me introduce you to Calabria</u>

The word "Calabria" comes from the ancient Greek word "Calab", meaning dense forest of pines trees. The pine trees still remain in the forest, located throughout Italy's most southern mainland province. They stretch down to the vivid blue sea, which cuts along a variety of beaches that can consists of fine black or white sand, large, polished smooth multicolored rocks or fine black pebbles that glisten like diamonds in the hot afternoon sun.

There is an abundance of history, art, architecture, culture and food that is difficult to find in Rome, Venice or Florence. Until a few years ago, what people ate in Calabria was different from what many English visitors were maybe used to. The Calabrese diet consists almost exclusively of pasta, pizza, fish and spiced sausage. It was virtually impossible to find Asian or other European cuisine in Calabria. Today it's different; in each supermarket now you see an Asian and other European cuisine sections.

The difference between the foods served in the north Italy to those in the south is that Calabria it is a lot spicier than you might expect. There are delicious wines to enjoy with your meals made in Calabria and other parts of Italy, and even in France. In Calabria you can enjoy the homemade liquors such as Limoncello the Calabria, made from lemon skin and citron liqueur. There is also Nocino, made from walnut skin. This is brown in color and highly aromatic.

The culture of Calabria also involves fishing along the shores. The Mediterranean is rich in tuna, anchovies, Muller, bass and clams. The most expensive fish is the neonata (Bianco Mangiare). The neonata is a special fish for making soup, and can be fried with a batter made with flour, water, eggs, grated cheese, a of pinch salt and black pepper. Spoon it into hot oil and fried it until golden brown.

Sheep, goats and pigs are very important to the farmers of Calabria. The goats mostly provide milk for many special Italian cheeses such as mozzarella, buffalo, casciocavallo, casciotte, fresh and dry ricotta cheese and pecorino cheese.

Life is conducted at a slower pace in Calabria; there are specific times to eat, to relax, to do business and socialize. You will find the rhythms of life as you explore your way through the towns, ruins, forts, forests, foot-paths, churches and historical centers. You will see sunsets offering viewers a light cast by the clearness of the atmosphere. There is one thing, if anything, that you will never, ever forget: that is the color of the water.

The Calabrese are generally very welcoming, helpful and traditional people. You may or may not understand the words coming out of their mouths, but you will certainly understand their gestures, their generosity and warm hearts.

The coast of Tropea welcomes any one to LA BIANCA SPIAGGIA (White Sand Bay) with an exclusive structure built by the sea that overlooks the entire coast. Both Mediterranean flora and exotic flora from tropical countries surround the complex. The white sand in the bay contrasts against the clear blue sea with magnificent seabed and abundance of marine fauna.

The Aeolian Islands stand out on the horizon, and the sight of Stromboli with its wisp of smoke can be admired every day. The natural beauty which surrounds it and the comfort of its furnishings make the LA BIANCA SPIAGGIA complex a unique place for a peaceful holiday by the sea.

Calabria is a land of ancient magic, generosity, tranquility and beauty. It will rejuvenate your senses and feed your eyes with a feast of colors. Calabria is Italy's best kept secret and yours to discover and appreciate in all of its beauty and all of its glory.

Calabria's has five districts: Cosenza, Catanzaro, Crotone, Vibo Valente, and Reggio Calabria. The district of Catanzaro is a province of Calabria and is one of the most interesting geographic places of the entire Italian peninsula. There is only 35 km between the Ionic Sea from the Tirreno Sea. From the mountains that face the isthmus, it is easy to compare the blue of the two seas and enjoy the dawn of the sunsets where the sun rises and finishes one's daily course from the water of the sea's rich history.

In the late 19th and early 20th century millions of Calabrians came down from their mountain redoubts and clamored onto ships that took them to "new worlds", particularly the USA and Canada. Today Calabria is different from the 19th and 20th century Calabria. Calabria is reclaiming its past glory and pride. When you come to the new Calabria you will be dumbfounded by its scenery whether you stay up in the mountains, or find your way along the winding coast highways that fall into Calabria's seaside towns and beaches.

You will find resorts, hotels, inns, bed and breakfasts, campgrounds, lidos and tourist parks. And once you've arrived and settled in, you will have the opportunity to savor the hearty, tasty, Calabrese cuisine, all made from local produce, meats, fish and fruit.

The district of Cosenza is quite a property. It is considered the most interesting of cultural and historical destinations. Paola is the synthesis of the great religious fervor of the Calabria people. Here there is the San Franceso the Paola Sanctuary, patron Saint of Calabria and of sea folk.

The young district of Vibo Valente has two centers: the hilly and the sea district with their respective ports, from which you depart to the summer connection with the Eolie Isles.

The district of Crotone offers occasions of historical reflections and landscape that brings us the splendor of the Magna Grecian. One km from Crotone is Capo Colonna, one of the most diffuse symbols of Calabria.

In the big district of Reggio Calabria remains one of the best known National museums. The district is rich in anthropology elements that unite in harmony the natural landscapes and place of history. From here to Messina, the first City of Sicily, looks like one can still touch, with their hands, the entire length of Calabria to Messina, with the beautiful waters in between.

Calabria's peninsula is narrow and approximately 250 km long. In all 5 districts, there are 402 cities and towns.

The History of Southern Italian Immigrants

Southern Italy has the most number of migrants to leave Italy. Can you imagine what it was like to say goodbye to your family and friends? To leave for a strange country, not knowing the language, and not having any money? Who would do such a thing? Why would anyone do something so drastic? The following is not a pretty story. However, it is a story that ends well, and needs to be told to make sure new generations do not forget what it was like for our grandparents, and what it was like when they got here.

When I came to America in 1968, everything was easy. Yes, I had to work but so did every other person in the country. My grandfather often told me about all the heavy labor he had to do when he come to America in 1911. He lived in West Newton, MA about seven miles from Boston. He walked to the city every morning, with 40 pounds or more of coal on his shoulders, and went back to Newton by 10:00am in the morning.

My grandfather said that he and hundreds of other men had to work in an open ditch, under a boiling sun, stripped to their undergarments. They toiled silently with shovels and picks. The

Greeks and the Southern Italians, however, who lived by selling fruit from the push carts in the city streets, earned considerable sums of money.

One by one they saved up for their sons, daughters and wives. If they had a son close to the age of 20, the father would appoint him first in line so that it would make it easier to have the whole family follow after him.

The immigrants who came in the late 1800s and early 1900s were faced with overwhelming prejudice, poverty and isolation from being in a strange and unfriendly land. I used to ask my grandparents why they never went to school. They told me that when they came to America they had to work and hope for a better life. They had to learn to adapt to the inconveniences that came before of us. However, they still held their heads high and were proud of where they came from and who they were. As the time went by, they learned to speak English, found better jobs and some opened their own businesses. Some joined the union and others bought their own homes. They succeeded in spite of prejudice, discrimination, and a less then friendly welcome.

I never forgot what he said to me. "We immigrants, we are only uccelli di passaggio" which means (Birds of Passage). Most Italian immigrants never planned to stay in the US permanently, since their intent was to be migratory laborers.

About 75% of Italian immigrants were farmers in Southern Italy. Many Italian men left their wives and children in the hope of returning back home (and many did and many more did not). In any event, for many Italian immigrants, migration could not be interpreted as a rejection of Italy. In fact, it was a defense for Italian work: to make money to be sent home, to help preserve the traditional order.

Rather than seeking permanent homes in the US, they desired an opportunity to work for (relatively) high wages in the city and save enough money to return to a better life in Italy. This was very commendable considering the difficult living conditions in Southern Italy during those times. These conditions were a result of many difficult factors. For us Calabrians, the vast majority of immigrants also came from Sicily, Abruzzi, Puglia and Naples, and Greece.

When I came to this country I saw all the improvements after what my grandparents had described to me. Of course, I came 56 years later. In my time here, I saw all the Italians stick together and even manage to preserve the Italian way of life. Today in the US, Italians mobilized to preserve their culture. In Italian neighborhoods you see Italian shops and other businesses open up. Italians made it a habit to buy from other Italians and kept the money in the community.

The time went by, you started to see Italian newspapers, Italian radio stations, and in the last century, an Italian TV station. Immigrant-aid and fraternal societies were formed. Sons of Italy are now all over the U.S. Each province of Italy is represented by societies in the U.S. Many Italian schools have opened all over this country. The biggest school that opened in the U.S. is the **Dante Aliguieri School.** Many societies formed from each Italian region where they also managed to have an Italian school which may only meet for weekly Italian language lessons. This helps our new generations keep our language alive.

After fifteen years in this country I became a citizen. What a day this was for me! For the first time I felt I belonged here in this beautiful country. I am very proud to say this today.

MY STORY: I AM AN ITALIAN AMERICAN.

Like many immigrants, I work and try to better myself as the years go by. 18 months after arriving in the U.S.A, I attended hairdressing school. I went to school eight hours during the day and worked 4 hours at night. In the beginning, it was hard for me because I did not speak English. I ordered four books from Milan, Italy called *Il Polyglots Modern* from Mondador Publishing. There were three sections in Italian and English on how to read and pronounce the English language.

At the time I opened a beauty shop in my home and worked for 7 years. I closed the beauty shop and opened a linens and giftware store. I worked until I became ill with severe asthma, in 1967.

I came to this country at age 26 and married my husband Peter at the age 28. We have two children, Alberto and Silvia, and three beautiful grandchildren. As a young girl I enjoyed cooking with my mother. At age 62, I published my first cookbook called *SAPORI DI CALABRIA, A Taste of Southern Italy.*

My recipes have been in my family for many years. Now I pass them down to my children and grandchildren. This book is organized into 3 sections. The first section I introduce to you the beauty of southern Italy and its history. The second section I describe to you my life with asthma for 18 long years and the impact it has had on my life and the life of my family. It would be hard for me to put on paper all the sick days I spent with asthma. The third section I added 80 of my best recipes for you to make and enjoy.

In writing this book, I hope to share my experience and help or save a life. Then I would say "Mission accomplished!"

Sometimes when I close my eyes I hear the sound of the ambulance sirens. I see how my husband and children are scared for me. Life with asthma has been a long and hard road for my family and I. When you have asthma as I have had for so many years, you are not alone in your suffering. Your family also suffers deeply.

One year in 1986, I was sick with the common cold, having also a cough and bronchitis. My crusade started in the fall of 1988. It started in September and for three months my family, doctors and I were all exhausted. The doctor sent me to do allergy tests. Soon after the new doctor saw me and before running any tests on me, he said "Mrs. Fusco you have asthma".

The asthma was so bad that the doctor started me with 60 mg of Prednisone per day, 200 mg of Theo-Dur three times per day, and "Theophylline", a not-so-distant cousin of caffeine. Imagine taking or giving your asthmatic child a caffeine-like substance just before bedtime to help maintain comfortable breathing overnight! At the time I have to inhale anti-inflammatory medicines. Now, it is rare that a patient needs more than 2 inhalations twice daily to keep asthma under control.

I became sicker and sicker instead of getting better. In February 1988, I was admitted to Newton-Wellesley Hospital from February 1 to April 1. I was admitted 5 times, almost 10 days to 2 weeks at a time. My primary care doctor made another attempt to help me and sent me to a pulmonary specialist. I was under this specialist's care for three months, but there was not much improvement.

My pulmonary specialist went to doctor's convention and spoke with my current pulmonary specialist for a second opinion. His name is Dr. Christopher Fanta. Fortunately I was very lucky to see Dr. Fanta at Brigham and Women's Hospital in the same week, after being discharged from Newton Wellesley Hospital after 2 weeks of hospitalization.

From 1986 to 1988, I was admitted to Newton Wellesley Hospital 14 times, having only a few times in and out of the emergency room. The day Dr. Fanta saw me he admitted me to the hospital and it was not until 14 days later my asthma was in control. I was hospitalized at the Brigham four more times until December 1988.

If you read my medical record, it says severe asthma with chronic bronchitis and chronic Prednisone use. Until 1995, I was hospitalized just for the asthma approximately 30 times. I do not like to remember those years of my life. I had two small children, and a blind husband to worry about at home.

In those years, every time the ambulance came to take me to the hospital, my husband said to the paramedic, "Please take my wife to Brigham and Women's Hospital. At times they would say no because I had no air in my lungs.

Many times I feared I would not go home from the hospital nor see my beautiful children and my husband again. All these years I spent most of my time taking Prednisone and multiple antibiotics. I became overweight in three months, gaining 30 pounds from 158 pounds. I became 205 pounds in no time. I felt very insecure about myself and what my body looked like, especially when people would tell me how much weight I put on.

They do not know what Prednisone does to your body and your life. But on the other hand we need to breathe and avoid having so many respiratory infections. If you take steroid at low doses, the risk is very minimal. I had to take very high doses of Prednisone over the course of 10 years. When I became so sick I knew about all the side effects I would have.

When my doctor became concerned about living a normal life, without too many complications, I knew there was no answer. So far the only medication that can treat severe asthma is steroids.

Steroids, when taken systemically, will restore our breathing capacity. We need to take our medicine and deal with the side effects as they occur. I have to take medicine for my stomach, such as Zantac, Pepcid, and for the last few years Prevacid.

In February 1988, I was in and out of Newton-Wellesley Hospital for three months and my primary care doctor ran lung tests on me. For one test, I had to keep a tube through my nose going down to my stomach for 24 hours. The test came out positive. I had severe gas reflux disease, (gastro esophageal reflux disease) or GERD for short. This means I had sensations burning in my stomach, sour taste in my mouth, and a hoarse voice.

From what I have read, the combination of acid reflux and asthma make asthma symptoms worse, especially at night. I had to elevate my headboard four inches to avoid the stomach contents rolling up, leading to a bad taste in my mouth. Acid reflux can be mistaken easily for symptoms of asthma. Without any doubt, I believe if you have asthma and GERD, when you treat GERD, your asthma will feel better and will protect your lungs from possible harm. You can treat GERD by modifying your diet and most of all modifying your portions late at night.

You can reduce your swelling by keeping your salt intake down. In the introduction of my cookbook, *SAPORI DI CALABRI*, I talk about how to reduce salt use. If you cook with lots of spices, you don't need to add extra salt in your meals. This will also keep blood sugar levels down. High levels of sugar are another side effect from long-term use of steroids. It is very important that we stay away from a lot of salt and sweets.

They are so many ways to improve our lifestyle if we take steroids for a long time. Another approach when you start to gain weight is to ask your pulmonary specialist to introduce you to a dietician. They will work with you to try to maintain your proper weight.

I know that the life for asthmatics is not easy, but the more you know about asthma and its treatments, the better choices you will make in caring for your own life and your children with asthma. It is a good feeling to understand what is going on in your body, to know how to respond to the signs that your body sends, and to breathe better again as a result of those actions.

My intentions for writing this book are to share with you the knowledge and the skills I learned from Dr. Fanta. I also want to help you understand asthma and to work with your doctor so you can plan to be in control of your asthma. I want to help you build confidence and a greater sense of security rather than feeling frightened by asthma.

Never feel embarrassed about asking questions. When you make a call for your appointments, talk to his or her secretary. You need extra time for your next appointment. You need to ask a few extra questions about you asthma. The doctor is there to help us in any way they can.

In Massachusetts, it is very likely that we have the best allergists and pulmonary specialists at the Brigham and Women's Hospital in Boston, especially for asthma clinician care. This is because of the long history of collaboration in asthma research. In 1989 Brigham and Women's Hospital formed a partnership called **Partners Healthcare** with Massachusetts General Hospitals. Over the years additional hospitals have joined the **Partners Healthcare** network including asthma specialists at Faulkner Hospital, Newton-Wellesley Hospital, and North Shore Medical Center.

According to the **Partners** Asthma Center's mission, this group of allergists and pulmonary specialists have one mission: to provide optional medical care for people with asthma and related diseases, to develop new knowledge about asthma and its management through state of the art medical research, to train medical students and graduate physicians in the specialized skills of asthma care, and to promote improved understanding about asthma and related diseases through educational programs and materials for their patients.

I am one asthma patient who has been so lucky to have known the most dedicated pulmonary specialist from this brilliant group: Dr. Christopher Fanta. You can reach any of these specialists directly at asthma@partners.org and visit their web site at www.asthma.partners.org or call 1800-9-PARTNERS.

Throughout the Asthma section I will provide you with the asthma emails and different telephone numbers if you need to use them. Feel free to get in touch with any of them if you need help! I am not a doctor or a nurse, but a person with a chronic disease called asthma, as well as a patient asking many questions in the doctor's office who has learned from it. Please consult your doctor for medical information as this book serves only as informational purposes. Any medications or treatment should only be taken under medical care from a physician.

ASTHMA

A long time ago, I asked my pulmonary specialist what is asthma. I remember it like it was yesterday. Asthma is a lifelong chronic disease of the airways in the lungs, with two important components: **constructions and inflammations.** These two components cause narrowing of the airways, which results in symptoms such as wheezing, coughing, chest tightness, and shortness of breath. They are also called asthma flare-ups or asthma exacerbations. I have had them all.

Inflammation is the swelling and irritation of the airways in our lungs. Airway inflammations are always there, even when we are not having symptoms. Asthma is a lifelong condition. But once we have taken some steps to help manage it, we may have more days without the asthma symptoms like wheezing, coughing, chest tightness, and shortness of breath.

I hope that my life with asthma will help others to take this disease seriously and learn to minimize asthma triggers and live a more normal life. We can learn more each time we go to the doctor's office, or read news from the Internet. After all, WE ARE BREATHLESS NOT HELPLESS! We need to remember to pace ourselves and consult our doctors before starting any type of exercise program.

I can never forget one time my son was 18 years old and I was very sick. Before he went to bed he came in my room and said hi to me. "Mom, call me if you need me at any time." At 2:00 a.m., I became very sick and my husband said to me, "I am going to call Alberto or else he would get upset if we do not call him." My husband Peter also told our daughter Silvia, "We are going to the emergency room at Brigham and Women's Hospital." We were near the hospital when I started to choke. I'll never forget that moment for as long as I live. My son went to pass another car in the road. He was very worried about me at the time and would do anything to get me to the hospital in time and it almost cost him his life.

Please never take severe asthma attacks for granted, never put your life or the life of your loved ones in the same situation I put my son. **ALWAYS CALL 911.** My asthma was triggered from dust, cool wade, cigarette smoke, paint fumes, and cat and dog hair. In my experience, even if your child does not have all of these allergies, it does not matter; all of what I state about can trigger asthma. So it is good idea to keep your child away from all of it.

When you go to the asthma specialist office, pick up books they have on display, in the sitting rooms. The TV and videotape you can also watch while waiting for your appointment. Everything they have on display that is asthma related, take home and read it together with your family. Everyone needs to know what to do in case of any emergency for a family member with asthma.

Asthma is disease of the bronchial tubes of the lungs. We need clean air to breathe. Curtains collect the most dust in you room, so wash them frequently and wash your bed sheet at least once a week or more. Cover your mattress, your pillow, and change your pillow once or two times a year. Stay always from wall to wall floor carpets.

If you have experienced asthma, you probably have a pretty good idea of what this disease does to you: coughing, wheezing, shortness of breath, tightness in the chest, itching under the chin, an uncomfortable awareness of your breathing, "noisy cats", and those of us with severe asthma we all know that panic attacks come very easy with severe asthma attacks.

To me, asthma came with every possible symptom: inflammation of the bronchi, severe coughing, which caused my ribs to fracture at one time or another. There were also huge amounts of inflammation, bronchial infections, and sometimes a fever.

Sometimes we want to know more about how our asthma is doing than just how we feel. With peak flow meters we can measure our breathing. The faster the air can exit from our lungs, the less active is our asthma. The slower the air is exhaled, the narrower the air passageways in our lungs become and the worse our asthma.

Having asthma puts us at risk for episodes of narrowed breathing tubes and difficult breathing. These are asthma attacks. With a peak flow meter we can measure how serious an attack is.

PEAK FLOW

Every person's best or target peak flow varies. When I was cleared from asthma and pulmonary infections, my peak flow always was 450 to 475. When my peak flow started to go down to 280, I knew I would get sick again.

If you have asthma you must know how the peak flow test is performing. I always repeat the test, than add 2 additional times. Then I record the best of the three tries. Then I will call my doctor and give him the best result I recorded.

In the beginning I was very uncomfortable with peak flow meters. They came in different shapes and sizes. I said to myself "How can I depend on this little toy to manage my air in my lungs?" Well the little toy makes me feel very good when the numbers reach 400 and over. The cost of peak flow is about $20.00. Often the Asthma Center will provide the patient with one free of charge.

Sometimes we, as patients, rely on doctors to do all the work to make us feel better, but this is wrong. As patients, we need to get involved and learn more about our treatments and our medications.

We need more campaigns, more people involved, more research for this disease. We need your help and patients, such as myself, to further involve themselves in this crusade.

My asthma is much more in control today then it was five years ago. But do not be fooled. Prednisone makes me breathe but deteriorates my bone. Your bones become very thin. I had to have 9 scopes placed in both my knees, all my ribs were fractured at one point or another with a cough, or just turning from one side to the other. Also, Prednisone causes severe attrition, stenosis, and scoliosis.

We all know that when we take inhaled steroids for a long time it still remains safer to use than regular use of oral steroids, such Prednisone. Prednisone has an increased risk of cataracts and glaucoma. I know because I am a living proof of this.

I developed cataract in both my eyes and had to have surgery. About 3 years ago, one night around 2am in morning, I started to have severe pain in my left eye. The only thing I saw in the eye was a big white round cercal. My husband called 911. When the paramedics came they said "This sounds as if you have a very bad head cold".

My husband and I insisted that the paramedics take me to Mass General Hospital in Boston. Soon after the doctor in emergency room saw me, she said to us, "It was good that you came quickly to the Hospital". My eye pressure was 33. I had glaucoma. If we did not insist on taking me to the hospital for few more minutes, I would have lost my left eye. Therefore, when we have severe asthma and take all the steroids, you are likely to get cataracts and glaucoma.

At this time, I was taking Asthmacort: 4 puffs in the morning and 4 at night. Most likely I was taking Prednisone too. When we want to get better, we need to take our medicine without worrying about the consequences.

It is very important to be aware about steroids and their side effects. As of today, I rarely have asthma attacks, and I thank Dr. Fanta for answering all of the questions I had and helping me to take care of and manage my asthma.

We need to have a plan to deal with our asthma and proper treatment. It is very important to work with your pulmonary specialist. Never stop taking your asthma medications without your doctor's approval! I still take medicines for Asthma, but very infrequently.

We all know that when we take Prednisone or another steroid for asthma, we need to decrease the dosage graciously as our doctor prescribes. Never stop steroid usage at will; this can lead to serious danger. Usually the steroids need to be tapped down every three days. We need to work to keep our circulations moving. When we take long periods of steroids, we can be rescued from blood clots.

Here are some quick remedies for treating asthma attacks:

1) Stay close to your inhaler. These quick-acting bronchodilators begin to work within 1-2 minutes. The most widely used, quick-acting inhaler is called Albuterol. It is available by brand name Proventil or Ventolin. When using inhalers, it is recommended to use it with a spacer to improve medication delivery, and always rinse your month after using an inhaler.

2) Take the medicine only if you have an asthma symptom. Inhalers don't need to be utilized if you don't have any symptoms. Use only as needed. I do not recommend taking quick relief medicine or over-the counter medicine for asthma. Some may have a few side effects. Is also good idea to consult with your doctor if you have asthma, before using an over-the counter medicine.

3) Have an asthma plan from your doctor. Together you will be able to create a plan for handling asthma attacks. I always know

that when I have an asthma attack my doctor or his associate is only a phone call away.

At this point my doctor prescribes me to take the right medicine, or call the pharmacy with new prescriptions when I need them. Severe asthma attacks can be dangerous. Always keep your doctor informed if you not are getting better. Seek help immediately by calling 911.

4) Ask your doctor for an asthma guide booklet. Usually they explain what you should do with a moderate or severe asthma attack.

BREATH OF FRESH AIR
Breath of Fresh Air: Partners Asthma Center is a news letter anyone can subscribe to.

Partners Asthma Center
Tower 4B, 75 Francis St.
Boston, MA 02115
Fax: 617-732-7421
E-mail: asthma@partners.org.

Pulmonary Specialist
Christopher H. Fanta, M.D.
Editor-in Chief
Breath of Fresh Air

This newsletter can clarify some of your questions and help keep you informed of new developments on asthma. If you visit this site, you will find different portions of information in various stages. Older issues of our Asthma Center newsletters, either in English or in Spanish, are also available. Descriptions of ongoing asthma resource projects from the Asthma Research Center are also obtainable.

When I look back I feel so fortunate, but not everyone is this fortunate. I want to explain to you the way it was during all those sad years of my life. I'm putting it on paper for anyone to read. I want people to know how asthma is a very serious illness and that it can be fatal if not treated, especially within children.

We hear about breast cancer, colon cancer, lung cancer and heart disease. Very little do we talk about asthma. As in my case, asthma can often be mistreated. You often can be treated for coughs, bronchitis, and then see only some improvement in the cough or no improvement at all.

Asthma is very easy to test and can be tested with a **pulmonary function test.** If your Pulmonary Specialist is located in an asthma center, pulmonary function tests can be performed at the doctor's office. With this test your doctor can see how the airway responds, and create your medication plan before leaving the office.

Today not as many children have asthma. Not as many parents need to learn about this disease. When children has a persistent cough for more a month, ask the pediatric to have you child test for asthma. I remember now when I was 9 or 10 years old, every time I was sick with a cough or bronchitis, my father would say to my mother, "Emilia seems to have cats in her chest."

Now I know what my father meant when he called the noise "the sound of cats in my chest". At age 46, I learned the proper name for it is wheezing.

No one had heard of the word asthma in southern Italy 55 years ago. When I started to have asthma attacks, I thought it came along with menopause. I asked my doctor if one gets severe asthma during menopause. The doctor could not confirm this because more research needs to be done.

I think if my doctor had conducted tests on me as a young child, I would have known I had asthma. My asthma would probably not have become so severe after all these years. I think back and cry because I feel guilty to have been in and out of the hospitals for so long. I feel that I have neglected my husband and children. I know that was not my doing. As wife and mother that was very hard for me to accept.

We need more funding for the **ASTHMA RESOURCE CENTER**. Doctors can do more research for this disease. We need to have parents recognize the signs of asthma so that early treatment can be started. Recognizing the signs and symptoms of asthma is an important part of managing your asthma.

VIRAL RESPIRATORY INFECTIONS

Viral respiratory infection was the type of asthma I had to deal every time my asthma occurred. If I came down with a simple cold and sinus infection, then I came down with viral infections, chest congestion, tightening across my chest and wheezing. Many a nights I lied awake sitting up or laying down on the recliner chair.

VIRAL INFECTIONS

Viral infections not only trigger severe asthma flare-ups, they also tend to make bronchial inflammation worse for several days to a few weeks. Asthma can become unstable due to increased bronchial irritability.

For most of us, the chances of avoiding viral infections during the winter months are slim. In those 10 years, I had to deal with severe asthma and viral respiratory infections every few weeks.

Living with asthma is not fun. Early treatment is most important. When I had severe symptoms—wheezing, coughing, shortness of breath, tightness in the chest—my peak flow numbers were under 280. This is the time to call your doctor's office and he will give you advice on what you should do next.

When I had the severe asthma attacks, my peak flow came down fast from 300 to 180. At that point you or a member of your family should call 911. There is no time to have a member of your family take you to any one of the hospitals.

Severe asthma symptoms are life threatening and a medical emergency. This means that the airways in your lungs have changed and that you need to go to the nearest hospital for emergency treatments. If you have severe asthma attacks that require urgent care in a doctor's office or emergency room of a hospital, you probably will be treated with nebulized bronchodilators.

Persons with difficulty controlling asthma may choose to have a nebulizer system at home rather than run to the emergency room. When I had to go to the emergency room, until the ambulance arrived, I would take some oral Prednisone as my doctor prescribed to me and start to give myself nebulizier treatment.

This would help make the trip to the hospital a little more comfortable. A nebulizer takes a liquid solution of medication and transforms it into a mist for inhalation. When I had the asthma attack, for so many years I used Proventil and Cromonil Solution. Today I only use Proventil medications, and maybe only 3 or 4 times per month.

Not everyone with asthma needs a nebulizer. If your doctor prescribes the nebulizer, your Healthcare Provider will help pay for some of it, and the other portion you need to pay as a co-payment.

Senior health benefits start at the age of 65. Medicare will provide a nebulizer and medications along with it for little or no cost, and deliver it free to your home. I know because my mother-in-law uses it and Medicare provides for it.

In the past I asked my doctor, "Can asthma turn into emphysema?" The answer was no. Emphysema is almost always due to cigarette smoking, or smoking related causes.

Cigarette smoking is another trigger that must be avoided. If you smoke, you need to quit. Smoking cigarettes will make your asthma worse, and if you breathe the smoke from someone else's cigarette, you may get an asthma attack.

Children are especially at risk when they breathe in secondhand smoke. Studies show that children of smokers are more likely to suffer asthma attacks, and their asthma will get worse over time.

But we can all do something about for this. We can protect ourselves, and our children and grandchildren. Asthma symptoms and asthma attacks usually are started by triggers. Find ways to avoid these triggers.

I am living proof what secondhand cigarette smoke can do. My father was a heavy cigarette smoker. When I was little girl I remember my father would get up from the bed during the night, sit up at the edge of the bed, and light up a cigarette. My father died from cancer, I have severe asthma, and my poor mother who never smoked, ended up having emphysema.

For your safety and your family's safety, please stay away from cigarettes. Life is too short to waste away with such nonsense! If you are parents, think about your children. If not, think about this for yourself.

TEENS AND ASTHMA

An asthma diagnosis does not have to define your teen. It is a chronic disease that needs to be taken seriously and treated appropriately. As a parent of a teenager with asthma, it is your goal to make living with asthma easier, but you should know that his or her need for freedom has to be balanced with treating the disease properly. If your teen only sees asthma as a disease that constantly limits their ability to do what he or she wants to do or what everybody else is doing, then treatments can become a major point of contention.

The key for parents is to give their teen some responsibility for their self-care instead of just giving them restrictions and limitations. Allow him or her to play a role in the treatment of personal growth with the disease. Then the disease will encourage personal growth and will help develop their self-confidence. Try to match the level of responsibility you play with his or her level of responsibility. Continue to play an active role in their asthma management plan.

They can participate in all facets of managing their disease, including the medications they take and the goals set for those treatments. As a parent you can talk to your teen about the consequences of not managing the disease, but trust your teen to take his or her medications at the correct time and in the right way.

Take a step back and allow your teen to take some control over his or her health. Remember to communicate openly, intervene when necessary, and talk to your healthcare professional.

CHILDREN AND ASTHMA

Parents are usually the primary care giver for their child with breathing problems. There are also often many other part-time caregivers in a child's life. They may need treatment while the other caregivers are in charge. Breathing problems can come at any time, so you want to be sure that everyone involved knows the right way to care for your child.

When your child has chronic breathing problems, there can be many challenges to your loving relationship. Treatment may be one of the biggest challenges you face. Children with asthma may be more fearful about the possibility of having asthma attacks at school, sports events, playgrounds, rather than at home.

Parents need to learn how to minimize their worries and those of their child, and to ensure that her or his asthma is under good control, at home, school, and at sports events. The best way to ensure this is to arrange a conference with your child's teacher and school nurse. Let teachers know how well your child copes with asthma, including inhaler usage and taking medications.

Sometimes a child will feel embarrassed about using their inhalers in front of other children and may worry that their asthma will prevent them from participating in a much-anticipated sport event or other school activities.

No matter how a good of a job you do in communicating your child's needs for quick access to her or his medication, at all times there may be asthma triggers for your child to contend with at school. You as parents will walk on solid ground if you ask the teacher to have animal hair removed from classrooms and carpets.

You hear sounds similar to a whistle when you child exhales. Or perhaps he or she seems to get easily tired when playing soccer or any other sport. Maybe there's just a persistent cough. But you wonder, could it be asthma? While asthma is a term often heard, it is frequently misunderstood. I of all people know this!

Asthma is, unfortunately, all too common. In fact, asthma is the most common chronic disorder in children and adolescents. 50 to 80 percent of children affected with asthma develop symptoms before they are 5 years old. I know this because my grandson is only 3 years old and he has been already been diagnosed with asthma at age 1. Because asthma affects the ability to breathe and to oxygenate the blood, it is a very serious disease.

The America Lung Association Unveils Kids with Asthma Bill of Rights

The Bill of Rights is a new tool created to help children assert their right to live active, healthy lives. The Bill of Rights is intended to start a conversation between children and their parents and parents and teachers. The American Lung Association is calling for changes about asthma and air pollution.

The Kids With ASTHMA Bill of Rights Contents

Statements that form the complete asthma management plan include the right to breathe clean air at home and at school, the right to play sports with a doctor's agreement, the right to effective and affordable asthma medications. The Bill of Rights also encourages children to work with their parents, teachers and doctors to create an **Asthma Action Plan.**

Children with asthma should expect nothing less than an active, healthy life free of frightening asthma episodes. A survey of school nurses conducted by the American Lung Association found that many school staff members lack awareness to the causes of an asthma attack.

Children, parents, and educators can visit the American Lung Association's Web site at www.lungsa.org to download the **Kids with Asthma Bill of Rights**. Parents, guardians or teachers can sign a petition affirming their belief that all children suffering with asthma are entitled to regular medical care and affordable medicines.

American Lung Association and Asthma

The American Lung Association created and funds twenty Asthma Clinical Research Centers throughout the country. They conduct clinical trials that provide important and immediate, practical information about asthma to help children manage their asthma.

According to the U.S. Environmental Protection Agency, air has been linked to the increased use of asthma medications, emergency room visits and hospital admissions by asthma patients. We all need to fight to have clean air both indoors and outdoors.

I do not want to see my grandson or any other child at his age take steroids. I am hoping to soon see new medications in the market for us, especially for small children. They need to grow up with strong bones and healthy joints.

But this is a disease that can be well managed. With a proper diagnosis, an action plan, and guidance from parents and caregivers, children with asthma can live their lives very similar to those of their non-asthmatic friends. Education and commitment are key for managing this disease.

Asthma can be a tricky disease to pinpoint for a number of reasons, including the fact that there are other respiratory ailments with overlapping symptoms, and some children can seem symptom free for long periods of time but then experience asthma attacks.

Children often miss school or daycare and parents miss their work due to their child's asthma. Clearly, asthma can have adverse impact upon the lives of many children and their parents.

Children who grow up in heavily polluted areas face an increased risk of continual asthma attacks. They are not as strong as adults to fight air pollution.

If your child has difficulty breathing in high air pollution areas, limit the amount of time your child spends outdoors and keep all activities as far as possible from roadways pollution. We also need to tell our Senator to defend any clean air acts. We need to work with the Senator to fight for clean air.

The only way we can achieve clean air for all of us and especially for the asthmatic people is for each community to be protected. Every American has the right to breathe clean air. If healthy people have trouble breathing in polluted air, how can people with asthma breathe normally?

Our children and grandchildren deserve a better deal than this. Our children need to grow strong and live a normal life even if they have asthma. If air pollution is the reason why we have an increased number of adults and children with asthma each year, we need to do something about it. We need to keep our air clean.

The Lung Associations has led the way for state laws and local ordinates that provide smoke-free public spaces to help people breathe clean air everywhere.

Allergies and Asthma

Allergies and asthma are common, serious, chronic childhood diseases affecting millions of children in the United States. In infants and children, asthma may appear as coughing, rapid or noisy breathing, or chest congestion. Proper diagnosis and management of childhood asthma requires a physician who recognizes the unique characteristics of childhood asthma.

With proper management and medications, an asthmatic child can lead a normal life. Watch for symptoms that can clue you in to seek the advice of a physician. This can include coughing (this could be constant or intermittent). Not all children who have this disease exhibit symptoms each and every day.

Wheezing or a whistling sound audible when your child exhales is another clue, as with shortness of breath or rapid breathing. This may or may not be associated with exercise.

Other symptoms of asthma can include fatigue that causes your child to slow down, stop playing, or become easily irritated. A child may have problems sleeping because of nighttime coughing or difficulty in breathing. Infants and young children who wheeze from viral upper respiratory infections also have problems sleeping.

Allergy: The relationship between asthma and allergies

This is a very individualized disease. The bottom line is to watch your child and then examine and test your child by a knowledgeable physician. It can make all the difference.

Asthma, a type of allergic disease, is a chronic inflammatory disorder of airways of the lung. Asthma is an ongoing disease; it requires ongoing managements and appropriate treatment. Properly managed asthma also includes using proper medications. Some of these medications should be used on a daily basis as instructed, even if you are feeling well.

If your asthma feels out of control, there are many steps you can take to make it better. Through careful detective work, you may be able to identify asthma triggers at home or at work. Doctor can easily discover whether or not your asthma is allergic asthma or a medical condition or caused by the medication you may take.

In my case for the first few months, I had to have injections for severe allergic asthma. This can be done in your doctor's office.

For children, exposure to allergens such as dust mites, mold, and animal dander can irritate their airways causing even more production of excess mucus and a tightening of the muscles that surround the airways. It is more difficult for children to detect these symptoms themselves.

Make sure you and your child follow your physician's instruction on the appropriate use and dosage of the prescribed medications. The better informed you are about your asthma triggers and management, the less the asthma symptoms will interfere with your activities.

Work with your physician on a management plan and take medications as prescribed. Together you and your physician can work to ensure that asthma does not interfere with your quality of life.

With seasonal allergies, if you have asthma, you may have a good sense when the pollen is count is at high levels. This may occur early in morning.

That means it is not a good idea to open the windows and doors in the house. Use air conditioning to cool your home. Remember when using air conditioning, it is important to wash the air condition screen every week or more.

If you or someone you love sometimes has trouble breathing because of asthma, and if you are inexperienced with asthma, you may feel powerless to help prevent the wheezing, coughing, or gasping symptoms that can appear to come out of nowhere.

My asthma symptoms were usually caused or triggered by a specific factor or combination including the following:

- Allergies to pollens, mold, pets, and other things in our every day environment.

- Air pollution such as tobacco smoke, traffic fumes.

- Emotions, including, fear and crying.

- Household irritants, including dust, cleaning products, and perfume.

- Medications, including some over the counter pain relievers.

- Weather, particularly wind and cold air. I know all about that.

I know as people with asthma, we cannot live in an allergen-proof bubble. We live complex lives with many competing demands on our time and energy. On the one hand, good breathing for our children and us is priority.

Anything we can do to improve our environment to help achieve our goal is desirable. Cover you month and nose with a facemask when cleaning your house, or ask your family member to do it for you.

All the chemicals and household cleaning products are dangerous for people with asthma, or for family members. Today they sell so many products in the store without ammonia, bleach and other chemical products.

REMODELING YOUR HOME

If you need some remodeling done on your home, during that time, go on vacation. A few years ago, when my asthma was worse, I had my floors refinished in my home. My family accomplished this job while I went to visit my mother. When I came back, my house was all done and I did not have to deal with paint fumes.

If the job is small, take day trips, and have your family member open doors and windows before you or your family members with asthma come back home.

When you remodel any room of your house, we all know what that means. We have to deal with plaster dust in the house and paint fumes. Later, we may find ourselves coughing and having asthma attacks.

Take this into consideration, even if you or your member of your family has asthma with no allergies, all these fumes can still play tricks on your asthma. We all know that fumes can be harmful even to a healthy person without lung disease. Never allow any one to bring into your home or in your car fumes of cigarettes smoke.

When I was in and out of the hospital, I put a sign on my front door. *No cigarette smoke is allowed in this house.* After that, if my guest wanted to smoke cigarettes, they had to go out in the street or in my back yard.

You and your family's health is your number one concern.

If some of your friends do not understand how fumes of cigarettes are harmful to you or your family, believe me: Their friendship is of no worth.

In my case I always had severe sinus infections. Smoke is another strong asthma trigger for me and for other asthmatics people. Sinus infections for me usually clear up with antibiotics. Most the time my sinus problem kept my asthma from getting better. Two years ago I was advised from an oncologist's doctor, a physician who specialized in sinus disease, to have surgery. I never had the surgery and this is another big problem for my asthma.

We people with asthma are number one in taking care of ourselves and our family members with asthma. It is no fun to live with this disease! Our goal is to have less coughing, less wheezing, less shortness of breath, and fewer awakenings overnight from asthmatic attacks.

The reward for these efforts: fewer symptoms of ASTHMA.

Although we cannot (yet) change our allergic sensitivities, we can reduce exposure to allergens at home and at our workplace.

No two people have exactly the same asthma symptoms; it's a very individualized disease.

I never take more medicine than my doctors prescribe to me. To do that is a very dangerous thing to do. So always consult with your doctor about your asthma. There are many things that can start up asthma and asthma can change, sometimes for better or for worse.

Often when I was improving, my pulmonary doctor needed to change my medicines, or new medicines may have been available at the time. I always have a big role in caring for my asthma. I see my doctor regularly. I keep in contact with my doctor to improve my asthma plan.

When you feel well and healthy, never stop taking your medicine. That way you avoid breathing problems from happening. Educate yourself about asthma: find out what triggers it and what you need to do to stay healthy. In fact, everyone in your family needs to know about asthma and know what to do.

Start taking control of asthma.

Learn your triggers and symptoms and what to do about it.

Learn what do to for asthma attacks.

Learn about your medicines so you know how quickly they should work.

Stay in constant touch with your asthma specialist.

Avoid your allergic asthma trigger.

During my illness with asthma, sometimes I needed to take anti-inflammatory drugs such as ibuprofen for attrition. Every time I would take this type of medicine, I had problems breathing. So my asthma specialist and I, we learned that I cannot take that medicine.

The bottom line is to stay close in contact with your doctor and especially when young children are involved with asthma. Watch your child and listen to their observations. If you suspect asthma, have your child examined and tested by a knowledgeable physician. It can make all the difference.

<u>Topics to Cover to at Your Child's Management Conference</u>

Your child's asthma history.

Medications delivery devices.

Asthma action plan.

Her or his allergies.

How to reach you.

How to reach the health care provider managing your child's asthma.

Plans for treatment when away from school, i.e. field trips, school sport events.

Ask your child's asthma specialist to send a letter to the school, describing your child's condition.

Get the most out of your child's visit to the doctor.

Learn all that you can about asthma.

Know when trouble starts with asthma.

Be ready to respond if the asthma gets worse.

Make good decisions about avoiding stimuli in your child's environment which he/she may be allergic to. Recognize signs of a severe asthma attack, and react to these signs as quickly as possible.

IMPORTANT THINGS TO KNOW AND DO

Exercise definitely induces asthma. Meaning, if you have asthma and exercise, you should never feel hesitant to call your doctor late at night in case of an emergency. A severe asthma attack is a medical emergency, and your doctor or another doctor is covering for him. There is always help in crisis.

After an asthma attack, we need follow-up care.

When asthma attacks are serious and require emergency hospital care, it is also necessary to follow-up your care with your Pulmonary Specialist in the office. You and your doctor can explore what may have caused your asthma attack.

Don't hesitate to take advantage of your follow-up visit, or any office visit. In collaboration with your doctor, you need to develop your **Asthma Action Plan,** and share some of information with family and close friends.

Ask all the questions you feel need to be answered about asthma. Doctors are there in the offices to work with us and make our life a little easier to cope with if stricken with asthma. Work with your physician on creating the most effective plan to keep you safe and healthy.

For me, the nebulizer treatment was the first treatment I used after having a case of mild or severe asthma attacks. Sometimes I needed to give myself two treatments, one after the other. With Dr. Fanta's plan, I always had steroid tablets (Prednisone). Taking steroids after having a severe or mild asthma attack is recommended, if directed by your doctor's plan. Later, call your doctor and let he/she know what happened with your asthma.

After I take the correct amounts steroid I am supposed take with Dr. Fanta's Plan, I measure my pick flow before calling him or the doctor on call. As a longtime asthma patient, we come to be our own caregivers for ourselves or our family members. Please never take severe asthma attacks onto your own hands.

Number one: We are not professionals. Number two: Severe asthma attacks never came upon me, even though it is very easy to have severe attacks and panic attacks (I call it a good marriage). I said this in the first pages of this book. When panic attacks occur, you feel worse than ever, and this can further complicate your health.

I always have my nebulizer next to my bedside and the phone. These two things are very important. Let a family member know where you keep all your asthma medications.

From the time I started having asthma until 5 years go, I was taking about 17 tablets from different medications on a regular basis. With asthma I had to deal with continuous sinus infections, gas reflexes, coronary disease, and severe attrition. And when you take steroids, depression comes very easily.

As of today, I take a one quarter of all those medications. I know when you have severe asthma, it is never going to go away. However, we can lead a normal life if and when asthma is under control.

I find the most important thing to do is to try and reduce stress when the asthma attack occurs. Breathe in and out, slowly and deeply. The physical therapist always recommends breathing 5 times very slowly and strongly.

This helped me to reduce the inflammation from my chest. Never take steroids without the consultation of your doctor. Communication between the asthma patient and doctor is the most important part of your asthma plan.

After taking steroids both in tablet form and intravenously while at the hospital, today I try to avoid decreasing the dose so I can avoid any serious side effects they may cause. However, remember that breathing is priority! It may be necessary to increase the dose of Prednisone for a time, and then decrease it again according to your doctor's plan for you.

While you wait for your breathing to return to normal, stay relaxed and breathe slowly and deeply. This will help your breathing return to normal and you'll feel more relaxed. In the beginning when I had asthma, I was in denial, and that gave me more trouble with asthma. Without the experience of having asthma, you can easily misjudge it, and the fear will always make your asthma worse. Relaxation is a very important part in managing your asthma.

Never leave your home without your medications. I have a small tablet box where I keep a few tablets of Prednisone.

Always keep your inhaler bronchodilator with you as well as your asthma physician's telephone number.

In 1992, I was coming home after doing my grocery shopping. It was in the winter months and halfway from home I started having breathing problems. It was getting worse after a few minutes and I was by myself in the car.

I stopped on the side the road and a police officer came by. I started to beep my car horn. He stopped, called 911 and I was taken to the nearest hospital.

I realized then I was allergic to cool wade. My asthma started in 1987 and after 3 years I was exposed to the fumes of paint. While I was at work, my boss called 911 and took me to the nearest hospital. I was so sick from 7 am until 7 pm. I started to get worse and finally starting feeling better at 7.30 pm. I was transferred to Brigham and Woman Hospital and I was in the hospital for 14 days. I never was allergic to the fumes of paint before.

We can define asthma in 4 steps:

Step one: Mild Intermittent.

Symptoms occur more than twice per week during the day and more than twice per month at night, with brief exacerbations.

Step two: Mild Persistent.

Symptoms occur more then twice per week during the day and more then once per week at night.

Step three: Moderate Persistent.

Symptoms occur daily during the day and more than once per week at night, affects activity and may last for days.

Step four: Severe Persistent.

Symptoms are continual during the day and frequent at night. Exacerbations are frequent and limit physical activity.

Step four details the history of my asthma for several years. My life consisted of frequent exacerbations, during the day and night. From one chronic inflammation to another, I had frequent office visits to my Pulmonary Specialist and was hospitalized many times. We can prevent some of this with our young children with new resources and new medicine.

Asthma can be fatal if mistreated. We can learn to manage asthma with appropriate therapies.

Children and teens with asthma miss more then 10 million school days annually, making this the leading cause for missed school days. When children miss school, parents miss workdays too. People with asthma have to be prepared at anytime. Anything can trigger asthma attacks.

I always carry with me my inhaler, my hospital identification number, my Pulmonary Specialist office number, and his beeper number.

When I had the allergy test done, the only thing I was allergic to was dust and cat hair but you can never know what attacks you when you have asthma.

With severe asthma, things can develop over time depending on where we are and what we are doing. It takes a long time when you have severe asthma to find out what things you are allergic to or not. Asthma comes in many forms such as bronchial asthma, allergic asthma, or in some cases, a cold.

We do not know why asthma comes in so many forms. In many cases asthma comes on strong during your middle ages. From what I understand, when asthma comes around during your middle age, it never goes away. Over time, it can get better or worse. I know my asthma will always be present and is never going to disappear.

So now I understand that my asthma is chronic. I have lived with asthma everyday. Some days are worse and some are better. As asthmatics, we need to know how to control our asthma and not let asthma control us. With a good plan from our doctors, we can live a normal life and enjoy our families.

CORTISONE DRUGS

I believe that someday we will have non-Cortisone drugs (Steroids) in the market. These medications reduce inflammation by minimizing swelling of the airways. Cortisone needs to be tapered down as your doctor prescribes. If suddenly discontinued, it can be vary harmful.

When the first doctor put me on a high dosage of steroids, my primary care physician sent me a letter and listed all the side affects from the Prednisone such as acne, increased blood pressure, dry mouth, bruising, leg cramps, hairiness, increased appetite, weigh gain, round face, cataracts, glaucoma, jitters, diabetes, muscle weakness, osteoporosis, depressions and weakening bones, and the list goes on and on.

When asthma is in control we do not need to take steroids, but as we know we always need to take other medications. For the last few years my doctor prescribed to me a new medicine (ADVAIR DISKUS). Advair helps control my asthma much more easily. It is easy to use and is devised with a built-in dose counter. You only need to take 1 puff in morning and 1 at night.

This is the reason why I started to write this book. We need to send a clear message to the research doctors. We deserve new medications in the market for asthma. But we all know that now is the time we must do more intense research. Doctors need more funding. With your help, we may have chance for a better life. With little funding and a lack of personal contributions, we have no hope for better medications. Doctors cannot perform research without our help. Our children and grandchildren need to grow up with strong bones and muscles. They deserve to live a normal life.

Thank you,

Emilia Fusco.

Send donations to:
Asthma Partner Center
75 Francis Street
Boston, MA 02115
Or call 1800-9PARTNERS

CONCLUSION

A doctor from **Partner Asthma Center** wants to train all medical students and graduate physicians in the specialized skills of asthma care: to promote, improve, the understanding of asthma and related diseases through educational programs for their patients, and for other health care providers and their community.

In conclusion, we need a prevention plan on how to control our asthma attacks. In our homes we do not have doctors around us and it is our responsibility to learn what we can use in our home and what cannot use.

EXERCISE

For years it was thought that asthmatics could not take part in team sports and vigorous activities. Today we know that is not correct. Exercise improves children, teens', adults' self esteem, and confidence. Not being able to do any exercise or participate in any activities can be a handicap for children and adults with asthma.

Today with proper detection, treatment, and a good doctor's plan, all people affected by asthma are capable of exercise that's beneficial to both their physical health as well as their overall well-being.

We need to learn about what triggers our asthma. In our homes, mold, dust mites, secondary smoke, and cockroaches can trigger asthma attacks.

Follow these steps to help control your asthma:

- Keep pets outside, if possible.

- Wash kids' stuffed toys and dry them completely.

- Mold grows on damp things such as shower curtains.

- Fix leaky plumbing as soon a possible

- Chemical irritants are found in some products in your home, including cleaners, paints, adhesives, pesticides, cosmetics, and air fresheners. All this can produce asthma triggers, particularly in a child. Use these products less often if possible, and make sure your child is not around when you use them. Also consider trying different products.

- Read all the labels whenever you clean a house: triggers are everywhere!

The following listed above can trigger asthma. When we have asthma, our immune systems are compromised and have difficulty defending us against the different substances present in the air we breathe in and out of our homes.

Asthma is an ongoing disease: it requires ongoing management and appropriate treatment. Proper management of our asthma also includes using the proper medications.

Don't let asthma manage your life; you manage asthma!

Discuss your asthma with your doctor and nurses. Keep a dairy of your medicine and learn what works for you.

Hospitals have support groups for asthma patients who meet monthly to share information and discuss ongoing issues.

I listed a few addresses and telephones numbers of resources in this book if you need additional help. If you live outside of Massachusetts, do not worry, every hospital in the United States has an Asthma Center for you to obtain the help you need.

<u>REMEMBER</u>

We are breathless, not hopeless!

Do not let asthma manage your life! You manage your asthma.

I hope that my work and my efforts in opening up my heart to you to write this book, does not go unnoticed. Please give us your HELP!

Thank you,
Emilia Fusco.

Send donations to the
Asthma Partner Center
75 Francis Street
Boston, MA 02115
Or call 1800-9PARTNERS

STARTERS, APPETIZERS & SNACKS

EMILIA FUNGHI RIPIENI
Emilia Stuffed Mushrooms

INGREDIENTS

2 dozen medium to large fresh mushrooms

1 pound Italian sausage (hot, sweet or your favorite)

2 tablespoons Italian parsley, chopped

2 tablespoons grated Romano cheese

½ teaspoon freshly ground black pepper

½ teaspoon salt

4 cloves garlic, peeled and minced

Pam cooking spray

DIRECTIONS

Preheat oven to 375F. Remove mushrooms stems and mince them. Brush the mushroom caps with lemon juice to prevent discoloration.

Remove the Italian sausage from casing and place in a bowl. Add the chopped stems, salt, and pepper and Romano cheese. Mix well to combine all the ingredients.

Spoon stuffing into the mushrooms cups and smooth into round shape. Place the stuffed mushrooms on a lightly greased baking dish. Bake for 10-14 minutes or until the sausage is no longer pink and the stuffing is golden brown.

Makes 6 servings.

<For a large party, double the recipe. Enjoy Emilia>

FACILE PIZZA APPETAISER
Easy Pizza Appetizers

IINGREDIENTS

12 oz fresh ricotta cheese

1 pound pepperoni salami, sliced into thin rings

1 package cocktail bread

1 ½ cup marinara sauce (see recipe in the book)

15 slices mozzarella cheese

DIRECTIONS

Slice pepperoni salami into 1/8 inch circles. Place half bread slices on a baking sheet. Top each slice with ½ teaspoon of marinara sauce.

Place 2-3 circles of pepperoni salami on top of each sauce covered slice, and cover with half slice of mozzarella cheese. Place under the preheated oven broiler for about 3 minutes, until the cheese is melted.

Makes 30 appetizer servings.

<Enjoy with your family and friends. Emilia>

MOZZARELLA DELIZIOSA
Mozzarella with a Twist

INGREDIENTS

1 pound mozzarella cheese

2 tablespoons pesto sauce (see recipe in the book)

½ teaspoon crushed red pepper

½ teaspoon dried oregano

½ teaspoon dried basil

DIRECTIONS
Cut the mozzarella into cubes and toss with pesto sauce. Sprinkle with crushed red pepper, oregano and basil.

This is the perfect centerpiece for a cheese platter. Each pound of mozzarella serves approximately 20 as part of an appetizer tray.

<Enjoy Emilia>

APPETIESE DI MOZZARELLA
Mozzarella Appetizer

INGREDIENTS

1 pound mozzarella cheese

Fresh basil leaves

1, 15-oz jar of sun-dried tomatoes packed in olive oil

1 head of lettuce

DIRECTIONS
Slice mozzarella ¼ to ½ inch thick. Top with a leaf of fresh basil and sun-dried tomato.

Serve on a lettuce leaf, sprinkled with the sun-dried tomato olive oil. Prepare two for each appetizer.

For a holiday accent, try cutting each slice into shapes using a cookie cutter.

<This can be fun. Emilia>

ANTIPASTO GOLOSO
Gulottas' Deli Antipasto

INGREDIENTS

1 head lettuce

12 marinated mushrooms

12 marinated artichoke hearts

12 green pitted black olives

12 black pitted olives

6 anchovies (salted packed Olive oil packed)

½ pound prosciutto, sliced

½ pound Genoa salami sliced

1 pound provolone cheese sliced

DRESSING

2 tablespoons extra virgin olive oil

2 tablespoons balsamic vinegar

2 tablespoons red wine vinegar

½ teaspoon dried oregano

2 tablespoon Italian parsley, finely chopped

½ teaspoon dried parsley

½ teaspoon salt

DIRECTIONS

Put all dressing ingredients into a small jar, close and shake well to combine all ingredients. Wash and tear lettuce into large bowl. Slice marinated mushrooms and artichoke hearts into quarters and olives in half.

Slice tomatoes in small wedges and chop anchovies. Cut meat and cheese into small pieces. Place all ingredients into in a bowl with lettuce, cover with dressing and toss gently.

Garnish with tomatoes wedges, olive and peppers.

<Buon Appetito. Emilia>

TACCHINO ARROTOLATO
Turkey Roll-Ups

INGREDIENTS

1 pound ricotta cheese

16 sliced oven gold turkey breast, sliced medium thick

½ cup chopped Italian parsley

½ cup roasted bell pepper, chopped

¼ teaspoon salt

¼ teaspoon freshly ground black pepper

¼ teaspoon paprika

In a medium mixing bowl, combine ricotta cheese, parsley, roasted bell pepper, and add salt, pepper and paprika. Spread each slice of turkey with 2 tablespoons of ricotta mixture.

Roll coated slices lengthwise. Serve whole or cut into pieces. Place on a platter garnished with green leaf lettuce and radishes.

Make 8 servings.

<Always double recipe for a large party. Have fun Emilia>

PROSCIUTTO COTTO E GENOVA SALAMI ARROTOLATI
Ham & Genoa Salami Roll-Up

INGREDIENTS

½ pound cream cheese

¼ pound Genoa salami

1 teaspoon Horseradish

½ pound cooked Italian spiced prosciutto

DIRECTIONS

In food processor, use steel blade to combine cream cheese, Genoa salami and horseradish. Spread each slice of cooked prosciutto with 2 tablespoons of cream cheese mixture.

Roll slices lengthwise and cut into 6 bite size pieces.
Serve on platter decorated with carved vegetables.

Makes 60 appetizers.

<From my party to yours. Emilia>

EROE ITALIANO
Italian Hero

INGREDIENTS

4 feet-long hero rolls

1 pound cooked ham

1 pound Imported Mortadella

1 pound Genoa salami

1 pound Provolone cheese

1 head iceberg lettuce

2 tomatoes, sliced

2 red roasted peppers, sliced

2 oz Italian dressing

DIRECTIONS

Cut rolls in half. Layer bottom half of rolls with all ingredients.

Place top half of rolls on top. Cut each sandwich in half

Make 8 servings

<Enjoy Emilia>

GORGONSOLA DI FORMAGGIO
Gorgonzola Cheese Ball

INGREDIENTS

1 cup cheese

1 cup of pistachios

1 cup of pecans

4 oz white Cheddar cheese

8 oz Gorgonzola cheese

4 oz light cream cheese, slightly softened, cut in ½-inch slices

¼ cup margarine, slightly softened, cut in 1/2-inch slice

3 tablespoons brandy, cognac, or cream?

DIRECTIONS

Position multipurpose blade in food processor. Add nuts, pulse 3-4 times; about 1 second each time, until nuts are chopped. Set aside.

With the food processor running, add shallot through feed tube.

Finely chop the shallot, about 5 seconds, scraping sides of bowl if needed. Add cheddar cheese: pulse 4-5 times, about 2 seconds each time until the mixture is crumbly.

Add the remaining ingredients; process until creamy, about 40 seconds, scraping down the sides of bowl if needed. Spread nuts on waxed paper. Spoon cheese onto a second sheet of waxed paper. Shape roughly into a ball with a rubber scraper.

(If too soft, refrigerate for ½ hour) Roll ball in nuts. Wrap and chill overnight to allow the flavors to develop. Serve at room temperature for best flavor.

Makes 30,1-tablespoon, servings.

<Have your children helped you. They will enjoy. Emilia>

IL RE DELLA COLAZIONE ITALIANA
Hot King Italian Sandwiches

INGREDIENTS

3 loaves of French bread

10 oz. Parma prosciutto, sliced

10 oz. Imported Mortadella, sliced

10 oz. hot Calabrian salami sliced (suppressata)

10 oz. Provolone cheese, sliced

6 roasted red bell peppers, seeded and sliced

3 tomatoes

3 cups chopped green salad

6 tablespoons extra virgin olive oil

1 tablespoon red chili pepper flakes

1 teaspoon dried oregano

INGREDIENTS

Cut French bread in half, horizontally. Layer one side of the loaf with all ingredients, one at time. In a small bowl, mix the olive oil, oregano and red chill pepper.

Sprinkle one tablespoon of oil mixture on each sandwich. Heat under the broiler for 2 minutes. Then, top the sandwiches with chopped green salad. Cover with the half bread and serve hot.

Makes 6 sandwiches.

<From the Italian Deli: to your table. Enjoy Emilia>

TORTARELLI IN CARROZZA
Calabrian Fried Sandwiches

INGREDIENTS

12 slices Italian bread (Scalia)

12 slices Provolone cheese

12 sliced Italian ham (prosciutto cotto)

4 eggs beaten

4 tablespoons milk

1 ½ cup bread crumbs

½ cup vegetable oil

DIRECTIONS

Top 6 slice bread with 1 slice cheese and 1 slice ham. Top with remaining pieces of bread and cut sandwiches in half to form triangles.

Beat eggs and milk together, dip sandwiches into mil mixture, then into bread crumbs. In non-stick frying pan heat oil and fry triangles until golden and light brown each side.

Do not over fry. Transfer sandwiches onto a dish cover with paper towels. This will help to drain the excess oil from the sandwiches.

Makes 6 servings.

<Enjoy Emilia>

EMILIA'S BRUSCHETTA

INGREDIENTS

6 roasted red peppers (see recipe in the book)

12 cans white cannellini beans, rinsed and drained

12 slices Italian bread

½ cup Marinara sauce

DIRECTIONS

Preheat oven at 375F.

Toast bread slices until golden, approximately 1 minute.
Transfer cannellini beans to a bowl: add marinara sauce and gently toss. Put the bowl in microwave and heat for 2 minutes.

Cut roasted pepper lengthwise and half inch wide. Lay half of the sliced peppers over the toasted bread and add 2 tablespoons of the cannellini beans. Serve when bruschetta is hot.

Makes 12 servings.

FOR RICOTTA BRUSCHETTA

INGREDIENTS

1 cup ricotta cheese

1 teaspoon fresh sage, finely chopped

1 tablespoon fresh basil leaves, chopped

½ teaspoon freshly ground white pepper

1 tablespoon extra virgin olive oil

DIRECTIONS

Mix all the ingredients in a bowl. Spread the ricotta mixture overreach sliced of bruschetta and serve.

This can be made 1 hour in advance. Refrigerate until your guests arrive.

<From my kitchen to your table. Enjoy Emilia>

FRITTALLE DI ZUCCHINI
Zucchini Patties

INGREDIENTS

36 Italian zucchini cut into 2 ½ inch pieces

1 small onion cut in 4 pieces

1 small onion cut in 4 pieces

½ small red bell pepper cut in half

2 tablespoons loosely packed Italian parsley

½ cup all-purpose flour

¼ cup fat-free egg substitute, or 1 egg beaten

½ teaspoon salt

¼ teaspoon freshly ground black pepper

¼ cup vegetable oil

½ cup non-fat sour cream

DIRECTIONS

Position reversibility slicing/shredding blade into food processor. Add zucchini and process until it is shredded. Remove the zucchini and place in a colander. Sprinkle with salt and let drain for 10 minutes. Squeeze dry.

Place a multipurpose blade into the food processor. Add onion, bell pepper, and parsley. Pulse 8-10 times, about 1 second each time, or until finely chopped.

In medium mixing bowl, combine zucchini, onion mixture, flour, egg substitute, salt and pepper. Heat oil in a large skillet over medium-high heat, until the oil sizzles. Add zucchini mixture by heaping spoonfuls: flatten with spoon.

Cook for 6 minutes, turn once or until golden and light brown. Transfer patties to a dish covered with paper towels. This will help drain the excess oil. Top the patties with sour cream.

(Variation: You can also sprinkle the top with confectioners sugar.)

<From my kitchen to your table. Emilia>

SALAD & DRESSING

MANGIARE LEGGER CON POCO SALE
Eat light with lower sodium

INGREDIENTS

5 cups Romaine or leaf lettuce

1 cup fresh mushrooms slices

2 small red onion, sliced

2 oz. lower sodium Bologna

4 oz. low sodium cheese

2 oz. low sodium ham

6 oz. turkey skinless, sliced

6 oz. no salt roast beef sliced

1 cup cucumber slices

1 cup asparagus blanched, and cut into 2-inch pieces

DIRECTIONS

Wash and drain lettuce and place in large salad bowl. Add sliced mushrooms cucumbers and sliced onion. Toss with julienne strips of low sodium Bologna, cheese ham, turkey and roast beef.

Decorate top of salad with slices of red pepper and asparagus. Serve with your favorite low dressing or vinaigrette.

<Have fun. Emilia>

INSALATA DI FRUTA
Citrus Salad

INGREDIENTS

3 large seedless grapefruit

3 large navel oranges

3 seedless tangerines

½ cup red raspberries

12 mint leaves

DIRECTIONS

Peel oranges, grapefruits and tangerines. Cut and section fruit to remove membranes. Do this over the bowl and let fruit sections fall into bowl, and then squeeze the remaining juice from the membranes. Add lemon juice and toss gently.

Transfer the fruit into 6 bowls. Divide the raspberries into equal portions and garnish each bowl with two mint leaves.

Make 6 servings.

<Enjoy Emilia>

CONDIMENTO ALL FRUTTA PER L'INSALATA
Citrus Vinaigrette

INGREDIENTS

1 ½ (12 oz cans) frozen orange juice concentrate, thawed

½ cup red wine vinegar

½ cup extra virgin olive oil

½ cup water

½ teaspoon freshly ground black pepper

DIRECTIONS

Add all the ingredients to a jar. Close and shake well. You can chill and store the vinaigrette for a week in the refrigerator. Let the vinaigrette stand at room temperature for about 15 minutes before using and shake well.

For a garlic citrus vinaigrette, add ½ tablespoon of minced garlic, or ½ teaspoon garlic powder.

For a ginger-citrus vinaigrette, add ½ teaspoon of fresh chopped ginger.

For an herbed citrus vinaigrette, add ½ teaspoon basil leaf flakes and ½ teaspoon oregano flakes.

All of these homemade vinaigrettes can be refrigerated for 1 week.

Makes 3 ½ cups of dressing.

<Have fun. Emilia>

EMILIA CONDIMENTO PER L'INSALATA
Emilia Condiments for Salads

INGREDIENTS

1 ½ cup extra virgin olive oil

1 cup red wine vinegar

2 cloves of garlic, peeled and chopped

1 teaspoon salt

½ teaspoon dried oregano flakes

½ teaspoon dried parsley

½ teaspoon dried basil flakes

2 tablespoons freshly grated Parmesan cheese

DIRECTIONS

In a jar with a tight lid, combine all the ingredients about, and shake well.

Refrigerate for 1 day before serving. Shake well before use.

This salad dressing can be poured over green salad and homemade potato salad.

<Make this in advance; it will save you time in the kitchen. Emilia>

INSALATA CON CARNE DI MANZO ALLE PESCHE
Beef & Peach Salad

INGREDIENTS

1 ½ pound top sirloin steak

2 tablespoons extra virgin olive oil

¾ cup lemon yogurt

½ cup freshly squeezed lemon juice

½ cup red onion, thinly sliced

½ teaspoon salt

½ teaspoon freshly ground black pepper

5 peaches, washed and sliced

DIRECTIONS

Rub steak with oil and sprinkle with salt and pepper. Grill steak over medium heat for 10 minutes, leaving lid open and turning steak halfway through cooking time.

For medium doneness, transfer steak to count a cutting board when a meat thermometer registers 150F. Let the steal rest for 10 minutes.

Combine yogurt, lemon juice, and red onion in a small bowl. If necessary, stir 1 tablespoon a lemon juice to reach a drizzling consistency.

Cut the steak, across the grain, into thin slices, and arrange with peaches on salad greens.

Drizzle the dressing on top.

<Buon Appetito. Emilia>

INSALATA DI PASTA
Pasta Salad

INGREDIENTS

12 oz. assorted colored short pasta, penne or fusilli

1 cup broccoli florets

1 cup cherry tomatoes cut in half

½ pine nuts

½ cup fresh basil leaves, cut in half

2 tablespoons Italian parsley chopped

½ teaspoon freshly ground black pepper

1 ½ teaspoon salt

1 cup green and red sweet peppers, sliced into 1 inch pieces

2 tablespoons salad dressing of your choice

1 tablespoon balsamic vinegar

DIRECTIONS

Cook pasta according to package directions. Four minutes before the pasta is ready to drain, add the broccoli florets to the pasta pot. Drain pasta when *al dente* and the florets are tender. Return pasta and broccoli to the pot.

When the pasta is cool, add all the remaining ingredients. This dish can be made for family dinner or a party. This pasta salad can also be made a day ahead. Just cover and refrigerate because the lemon juice will help all the ingredients to maintain their color.

Makes 4 servings.

<Have fun. Emilia>

INSALATA DI GAMBERI AL LIMONE
Tossed Salad with Shrimp & Lemon juice

INGREDIENTS

2 pound fresh peeled shrimp, peeled and de-veined

10 cups fresh mixed greens

1 bunch baby asparagus

1 15 oz can of artichoke hearts

2 tablespoon fresh basil leaves, chopped

1 tablespoon margarine

2 cloves garlic, peeled and minced

VINAIGRETTE

¼ cup white wine vinegar

¼ cup lemon juice

2 tablespoons lemon zest

2 tablespoons extra virgin olive oil

1 cup red onion, thinly sliced

DIRECTIONS

Trim asparagus and cut 1 ½ inch long. Blanch in boiling water for 2 minutes.

In a small jar combine all the ingredients for the vinaigrette. Cover with lid and shake well until blended and refrigerate for 2 hours or until serving time.

In skillet heat margarine and sauté garlic until golden, add shrimps and sauté until turn pink. Let cool for 5 minutes.

In a large salad bowl combine mixed salad, cooked shrimp, artichoke, and asparagus.

Pour vinaigrette over the salad and toss well. Serve cool for lunch or a family brunch.

Makes 8 servings. <Cook for your family and friends is fun. Enjoy Emilia>

INSALATA DI POLLO RISO & ARUGOLA
Chicken, Rice & Arugula Salad

INGREDIENTS

2 ½ cups of uncooked instant brown rice

4 boneless skinless chicken breast halves

¾ cup pine nuts

10 cups arugula

1 cup red and green onions, sliced

1 cup red and green bell pepper, seeded and thinly sliced

1 cup cherry tomatoes, halved

2 ½ cups chicken broth

1 ½ cups water

FOR THE VINAIGRETTE

1 tablespoon lemon peel

¼ lemon juice

½ teaspoon salt

½ teaspoon freshly ground black pepper

¼ cup extra virgin olive oil

2 tablespoon balsamic vinegar

½ cup blue cheese, crumbled

DIRECTIONS

Add the vinaigrette ingredients in a jar; shake well, cover and refrigerate for 2 hours or until serving time.

Combine water and broth and bring to a boil. Stir in the rice, cover and remove from heat. Let stand 5-7 minutes, and then fluff rice with fork.

Wile the rice is cooking and cooling; broil the chicken breast in the oven broil or an outside grill for 4 minutes on each side.

Cut roast chicken in small strips and mix in a bowl with the vinaigrette, then combine rice and vegetables in large bowl, mix well.

Add half the pine nuts and vinaigrette mixture. Transfer salad mixture onto a serving platter and garnish salad with remaining pine nuts. Refrigerate until serving time.

Makes 6-8 servings.

<Buon Appetito. Emilia>

I

INSALATA DI PATATE E MELANZANE
Potato Salad with Eggplants

INGREDIENTS

3 Italian eggplants

4 large potatoes

1 teaspoon fresh oregano chopped

4 mint leaves chopped

½ cup red onion, chopped

2 tablespoons extra virgin olive oil

2 tablespoons red? white? wine vinegar

½ teaspoon salt

¼ teaspoon freshly ground black pepper

DIRECTIONS

Wash eggplants and cut into pieces 1 ½" long by ½" thick. Blanch for 1 minute in lightly salted boiling water: drain eggplants and let cool of before mixing with the potatoes. Boil the potatoes for at least 30 minutes.

Peel potatoes, and slice them the same length of eggplants. Transfer potatoes, eggplants into a salad bowl. In a small bowl mix oil, vinegar, salt and pepper, oregano and mint.

Pour the vinegar mixture over potatoes and eggplants. Gently mix and serve cold. This salad can be prepared 2 hours before and kept in the refrigerator. For a large party, double ingredients.

Makes 6 servings.

<Have fun. Emilia>

INSALATA DI VEGETALI E TACCHINO
   Turkey and Vegetable Salad

INGREDIENTS

3 red, green and yellow peppers, seeded and cut into ½ inch strips

1 cup zucchini, sliced ½ inch thick

1 cup yellow summer squash, sliced ½ inch thick

10 cup mixed greens, torn into bite-sized pieces

6 oz Fontina cheese, cut ½ inch chunks

6 oz cut into ½ inch strips

1 cup cherry tomatoes cut in half

2 tablespoons basil leaves chopped

½ cup white onion, sliced

4 oz vinaigrette dressing (see recipes in the book)

DIRECTIONS

In a large bowl toss peppers, zucchini, summer squash and dressing. Remove with slotted spoon and reserve the dressing. Grill for 15 minutes or until tender, turning frequently. Return grilled vegetable to reserved dressing, cover and refrigerate.

While the vegetables are chilling, wash and spin dry the mixed greens. Cover the bottom of 6 salad plates with greens. Toss cheese and roast turkey with the grilled vegetables and dressing. Spoon the mixture onto the bed of greens. Garnish with chopped basil leaves.

Makes 6 Servings.

<From my kitchen to your tables. Enjoy Emilia>

SALSA AL PESTO DI PREZZEMOLO
Parsley Sauce

2 cups parsley, steams removed

4 clove garlic peel

½ cup extra virgin olive oil

4 tablespoons water

1 teaspoon salt

½ teaspoon freshly ground black pepper

DIRECTIONS

In a blender add all ingredients, except the water. Blend until smooth, then drizzle in the water 1 tablespoon at time if needed.

This sauce can be saved in a plastic container or in a jar with tight lid for 1 week or in a freezer for up 2 months.

<Making this in advance will save you time. Emilia>

INSALATA CON, FAGIOLINI E CIPOLLA
Steak Salad with Green Beans & Onion

INGREDIENTS

3 pound sirloin steak, about 3 steaks

1/2 pound fresh bocconcini mozzarella cheese

½ cup red onion, sliced ¼ inch thick

1 pound green beans, trimmed

2 head Romaine lettuce, cut into bite-sized pieces

2 tablespoons extra virgin olive oil

1 tablespoon white vinegar

DIRECTIONS

Coat steak with 1 tablespoon oil, season with salt and black pepper. Heat a large, nonstick skillet over medium high heat. Cook steak until browned, about 4 minutes per side. Transfer steaks to a cutting board, cover and let rest 5 minutes before slicing thinly.

In a large nonstick skillet heat 1 tablespoon oil and sauté onion until lightly golden. Add green beans to the skillet and ½ cup water: cover and cook until tender and brown, about 5 minutes, uncover and cook for 2 minutes long or until beans are browned.

In a large bowl, gently toss lettuce with half the dressing. Divide among 6 plates. Arrange beef, mozzarella cheese, and vegetables over lettuce. Drizzle top with remaining dressing and if needed, add more salt and pepper.

Makes 6 servings.

<Buon Appetito. Emilia>

INSALATA DI ASPARACI, ARANCI E ESCAROLE
Asparagus, Orange & Endive Salad

INGREDIENTS

1 ½ asparagus, trimmed and cut diagonally

2 cups rinsed, dried and torn endive leaves

2 large oranges, sliced into rounds

1 red onion, thinly sliced

1/3 cup raspberry vinegar

2 tablespoons extra virgin olive oil

1 tablespoon orange juice

1 tablespoon white sugar

½ teaspoon salt

¼ teaspoon freshly ground black pepper

DIRECTIONS

To a large pot of boiling water, add asparagus, endive, orange and red onion. Blanch for 1 minute: drain and plunge asparagus into a bowl of cold water. Drain again and dry.

Wisk together the raspberry vinegar, oil, orange juice, sugar and salt and pepper. Add dressing to the asparagus mixture, toss well and serve.

Makes 4 servings.

<Enjoy Emilia>

VEGETALI CON I SAPORI DI CALABRIA
Vegetables with a Southern Italia Taste

Salad and other greens: Southern Italy is the best land for greens. Almost anything that grows in garden can be used in risotto dish, minestrone, soups and salad.

Broccoli and Broccoli Rabe: these two vegetables are from the same family, but have very different tastes. Broccoli has a very mild taste and broccoli rabe has a bitter taste. Both can be boiled or steam.

Arugula: A green Mediterranean lettuce that can also be use in a risotto, pastas and minestrone soups.

Escarole: This green lettuce can be use in minestrones, salad and sautéd with beans.

Tomatoes: An important part of the Southern cuisine. Canned, whole, diced, crush, or purred they are use for sauce, soups, minestrone, pizzaiola and bruschetta.

When shop to by Italian tomatoes to make your on sauce. Look for Italia brands. (Pastine kitchen ready, Progresso, Rienzi and Contadina, crushed, or peeled tomatoes.)

Italian cooking would not be the same without tomatoes!

Oregano: Oregano is the most used spice in Southern dishes. Used to season pizza topping, tomatoes salad and sauces.

Sage: Used to flavor pork, veal and, lamb and others meats.

Italian parsley: It has flat leaves and more flavor than curly parsley. If can be used for Italian meatballs salads, cook meats and to garnish dishes.

Basil leaves: Fresh basil is a popular Italian herbs used to make pesto sauce, seasoned tomato salad, to flavor sauces and garnish dishes.

Onion: A delicious flavor when add to sauces, soups, minestrone salad dressing and meats.

Garlic: Used peeled, chopped or mince. In the Southern Italy; garlic is the number one spice used in food. When browning garlic, be very careful with the hot oil and always make garlic golden and light brown. If the garlic is burnt, discard the oil or you will have a burnt taste in your food.

Mushrooms: Makes favorite dishes like chicken and turkey into exotic dishes. Mushrooms are picked on our land and they come in so many names: Cauliflower, Porcini, Portabello, Oyster, Cremini, Shitake, and Chanterelle. They are so many varieties and they are sold at the market for a high price.

My Mother always preserves mushrooms. In the region I come from, preserving our farm produce is very important.

Pickled mushrooms can also be used in salads, antipasto dishes and pasta dishes and appetizers. They can also be cleaned and frozen up to 6 months.

Eggplants, zucchini and peppers; These three vegetables are used to make a complete meals. Can be stuffed, marinated, fried, used in minestrones, roasted pickled and used in salads.

The Italian tradition of combining herbs and spice is the best for adding flavor to your dish. On occasion you may not have fresh herbs in your kitchen; you can substitute dry herbs and spice: this will work just as well. Only use ¼ to ½ teaspoon.

When I cook for my self and family: I do not use salt, all the vegetables and spice; combined together will give me lots flavor without adding salt.

Imagine your kitchen filled with these beautiful aromas, flavors and spices. Cooking with love means enjoying your meals. Spices and vegetables can be preserved in the summer for the winter months.

You can create hearty, comforting meals in your kitchen that you and your family will enjoy more then going out to eat. You can choose your own ingredients, your own amount of oil and avoid butter and other fats.

Today you don't need a passport to test fabulous meals with the flavors from faraway lands like Southern Italy. All supermarkets and grocery stores are now filled with Italian herbs and spices.

<Thank you for joining me on this culinary adventure. Emilia

PEPPERONI, MALENZANI E ZUCCHINI SOTTO ACETO
Peppers, Eggplants & Zucchini in Vinegar

INGREDIENTS

3 large red bell peppers

3 Italian eggplants

3 zucchinis

3 cups white vinegar

1 ½ cup water

1 tablespoon salt

4 cloves of garlic, peeled and chopped

¼ teaspoon dried oregano

1 cup of capers

2 tablespoons olive oil

DIRECTIONS

Wash, core and seed peppers, then cut top and bottom from eggplants and zucchini; then slice the zucchini into long strips, about 2 ½ inch long per ½ thick. In a large saucepan add vinegar, water and salt.

Bring the mixture to a boil, add the vegetables strips and let them boil for 30 seconds. Drain using a slotted spatula and transfer into a colander for 1 minute.

Put the vegetables on a dish towel until cool and all the liquid is removed. Transfer the vegetables into a salad dish and add all the remaining ingredients.

Toss gently and serve. For preserving these vegetables. Spoon vegetables into a Mason jar: cover the vegetables with vegetables oil. Seal the jar and store in the refrigerator.

(These vegetables will make for a good antipasto next to cheese and salami dish.)

<This can be fun and enjoy good taste when you eat. Emilia>

PEPERONI ROSSI ARROSITE
Roasted Red Peppers

INGREDIENTS

6 large red bell peppers

2 tablespoons oil

2 cloves of garlic, peeled and chopped

2 tablespoons Italian parsley chopped

DIRECTIONS

Pre-heat broiler at a high temperature. Place rack in the oven, under the broiler, to roast the peppers. As the peppers begin to blister, use a tong to turn them over as each side should have an even blister. Let the peppers cool for 5 minutes, and then remove the skin and seeds.

Slice the peppers ½ inch thick lengthwise: lay them over paper towels to dry. Put peppers into a small bowl, add oil, garlic and chopped Italian parsley.

To freeze: Cut peppers into half. After the peppers are dried, put them into freezer bags. You can freeze them for up to 6 months.

Roasted peppers can be added to a pasta, bruschetta, and antipasto.

<Buon Appetito. Emilia>

VEGETALE ALLA GRIGLIA
Grilled Veggie Sandwich

INGREDIENTS

12 slices of Italian bread

4 cloves of garlic, crushed

1 Italian zucchini, sliced

1eggplant, sliced

2 large tomatoes, sliced

1 large red onion, sliced

1 yellow squash

1 large red pepper, sliced

1 yellow pepper sliced

1 red pepper sliced

½ cup crumbled blue cheese

1 teaspoon lemon juice

2 tablespoons olive oil

½ teaspoon salt

½ teaspoon freshly ground black pepper

DIRECTIONS

Preheat the grill for high heat.

In a small bowl, combine lemon juice, oil crush garlic and set sauce aside in the refrigerator. Brush vegetables with oil on each side; and brush the grill with oil. Place the bell pepper and zucchini closet to the center of the grill, and the remaining vegetables around them.

Cook for about 2 minutes and turn to the other side, only peppers and zucchini need to be on the grill a little longer. Remove vegetables from grill and set aside.

Spread the oil mixture evenly over 6 sliced of bread, and sprinkle over the blue cheese. Place slice bread all round on the grill and remove soon the blue cheese is melted. This will warm the slice of bread.

Remove from grill, and layer 2 pieces with roast vegetables. Cover with remaining slice of bread and serve warm.

(Optional) Add a pinch of crush red hot pepper if anyone likes spicy food.

<Enjoy Emilia>

ZUCCHINI AL FORNO
Baked Zucchini

INGREDIENTS

6 small Italian zucchini

1 cup whipping cream

½ cup milk

½ teaspoon ground fresh pepper

2 cloves of garlic, peeled and minced

½ cup great Parmesan cheese

1 cup Fontina cheese, shredded

½ teaspoon salt

Cooking spray

DIRECTIONS

Preheat oven to 375 F. and spray a baking dish with cooking spray.

Wash and cut zucchini into ½ inch rounds and let drain into a colander for 5 minutes, pat dry with paper towel to avoid excess moisture on the zucchini.

In a bowl combine cream, milk, minced garlic and black pepper and beat until puffy. Layer half the zucchini in the greased dish; top with half of the cheeses and half of the whipping mixture.

Repeat layer with zucchini, the whipping mixture and top with reaming cheeses. Bake un-covered for 10 minutes. The zucchini should be tender and the cheeses melted. Let it stand 4 minutes before serving. Serve with a side of rice or baked chicken.

Makes 4 servings.

<Buon Appetito. Emilia>

RISOTTO E POLENTA
RISOTTO CON ASPARACI
Risotto & Asparagus

INGREDIENTS

1 pound asparagus spears, trimmed

2 tablespoons extra virgin olive oil

2 clove garlic, peeled and chopped

2 tablespoon minced onion

4 cups chicken broth

2 cups dry white wine

1 pound Arborio rice

¼ teaspoon salt

¼ teaspoon freshly ground black pepper

¾ cup fresh grated Parmesan cheese

DIRECTIONS

Add asparagus to boiling water and cook for 4 minutes. Drain water from asparagus and set aside. While asparagus is cooking, add oil butter garlic and onion to a large skillet and sauté until garlic and onion are golden.

Add 3 cups chicken broth, white wine, salt and pepper. Cover and simmer at low medium heat for 10 minutes.

Keep stirring until the rice absorbs all the liquid and the rice is cooked.

Add half the Parmesan. Topping the risotto with asparagus and the remaining cheese. Makes 6 servings.

<Enjoy Emilia.>

RISO E VEGETALI
Vegetable Rice

INGREDIENTS

1 pound Arborio rice

2 pound cherry tomatoes cut in half

¾ cup pitted black olives

¾ pound pitted green olives

8 oz. washed and dried button mushrooms, cut and quartered

½ cup yellow onion, minced

4 clove garlic, peeled and chopped

3 tablespoons capers, rinsed

2 tablespoons chopped fresh basil leaves

2 tablespoons freshly minced Italian parsley

½ cup white wine (extra dry)

2 tablespoons extra virgin olive oil

½ teaspoon salt

½ teaspoon freshly ground black pepper

DIRECTIONS

Heat oil in a large saucepan. Add garlic and onions and sauté until golden brown. Add mushrooms, cook for 1 minute, and do not brown: add cherry tomatoes, olives, capers, basil leaves, salt and pepper. Cook for about 12 minutes: and stirring constantly.

Meanwhile in a large pot, boil lightly salted water. Cook rice according to package directions. Cook and drain rice *al dente* and add to the sauce mixture. Add the Parmesan cheese, stirring and garnished with chopped parsley. Serve hot.
Makes 6 servings.

<Buon Appetito. Emilia>

EMILIA POLENTA
Emilia's Cornmeal

INGREDIENTS

8 cups water

1 ½ fine cornmeal flour, (not quick cooking)

8 cups water

1 teaspoon salt

½ cup Parmesan grated cheese

DIRECTIONS

In a large saucepan, dilute 1 cup cornmeal flour and salt while stirring constantly. Gradually add the remaining flour and whisking until smooth. Set heat on medium-low and keep stirring for 30 minutes.

Reduce heat to low simmer; whisking often until thickened about 10-15 minutes long. Remove from heat: stir cheese in and serve hot. For thick polenta, add ¼ cup or more cornmeal flour in the beginning.

For a green polenta add three cups of chopped and washed broccoli rabe leaves into the water after dilute the first cup of cornmeal flour. Polenta can be served as first meal. With a spatula, cover a flat dish with polenta, add as a side to broiled meats or fish.

Polenta can be served in slices. If you have a wood surface, transfer polenta over and let it cool before cutting; flatten the polenta with spatula and use a knife to cut the polenta strips about 1 inch thick and cut 2 ½ inches long.

Brush any cookie pan with lightly with olive oil. Arrange slices in a single layer, and brush top with olive oil. Heat broiler: and broil about 4 inch from heat.

Broil for 5 minutes or until is golden and light brown. Polenta can be served with sauté mushrooms or a chunky tomatoes sauce.

Polenta with broccoli rabe: can be serving soft or cut and broiled. In the region I come from: polenta with broccoli rabe sometimes is served as an antipasto.

About 45-50 years go, polenta was the poor people's meal. Everyone grows corn and in my town cornbread was on everyone's dinner tables.

<Enjoy these meals with me. Emilia>

RISO CON FAGIOLI CANNELLINI AL FORNO
Cannellini Rice Bake

INGREDIENTS

1, 14 oz can of cannelloni beans

1 pound Arborio rice

1 teaspoon salt

½ cup Parmesan cheese, grated

2 ½ cups marinara sauce

DIRECTIONS

In a large pan, boil salted water and cook rice according to package directions. Drain and cook rice al dent. In the same pan mix rice and 2 cups sauce and half the Parmesan cheese.

In a large baking dish pour a half cup of the marinara sauce over the rice mixture. Sprinkle over the remaining cheese and bake uncovered in a preheated oven at 400 F for 20 minutes or until the top is golden brown.

(Optional) Mix the remaining cheese with 2 tablespoons of Italian flavored breadcrumbs and sprinkle over the top before baking. This will make a hard crust for the rice.

<Buon Appetito. Emilia>

ORANGINI DI RISO RIPIENI
Stuffed Fried Rice Balls

INGREDIENTS

8 oz. Arborio rice

½ cup Romano cheese

½ teaspoon salt

¼ teaspoon freshly ground black pepper

2 eggs beaten

1 ½ cups breadcrumbs

1 ½ cups vegetables oil for frying

FOR THE STAFF

½ cup cook peas

½ cup cooked ground pork in marinara sauce

½ cup shredded mozzarella cheese

DIRECTIONS

Cook rice in a large pot of lightly salted boiling water according to package directions. Drain rice *al dente* and let it cool in the colander.

Transfer rice to a bowl and mix in the Romano cheese, parsley, black pepper and the eggs beaten. In a small bowl, mix mozzarella cheese, peas and meat sauce. Drain any of the remaining liquid.

In a flat dish, add the breadcrumbs. With a spoon, take 1 spoon rice and put into the palm of your hand, make a hole in the center.

Add 1 teaspoon of the meats mixture and cover with rice. Make round balls and roll them into the breadcrumbs. In a pan heat oil until very hot and very gently add the rice balls one a time.

Fry them until golden and light brown all round. Take *orangini* out the fry pan with a slotted spoon to drain all the excess oil, and put them in a dish covered with a paper towel.

Transfer onto a serving platter Serve hot or cold as an appetizer.
<From my kitchen to your table. Enjoy Emilia.>

RISO CON POLLO E PISELLI AL LIMONE
Lemon Rice with Chicken & Peas

INGREDIENTS

14 oz. Arborio rice or Pastine

1 cup frozen peas, thawed

½ pound chicken breast, skins removed

½ teaspoon salt

¼ teaspoon freshly ground black pepper

2 tablespoons Italian parsley finely chopped

1 teaspoon margarine

2 tablespoons extra virgin olive oil

½ cup Asiago cheese grated

1 tablespoon lemon zest

2 tablespoons lemon juice

¼ cup extra dry white wine

1 clove garlic peel and chopped

DIRECTIONS

Heat the broiler and cook the chicken until it is no longer pink. With knife cut the chicken into small pieces and set aside. In a large pot of boiling salted water, cook rice according to package direction.

Cook rice *al dente*, drain and set aside. To a skillet add margarine, oil, sauté garlic until golden. Add peas, pinch salt, black pepper, wine, lemon zest and lemon juice.

Cook on low medium heat until peas are tender. If you need little more juice, add few tablespoons white wine.

Add rice and chicken to the skillet and half the Asiago cheese and sauté for 30 second to blend all the mixture. Transfer into a serving dish. Garnish with chopped parsley and remaining cheese. Serve hot.

Makes 6 servings.

<Buon Appetito. Emilia>

SALMONE E RISO
Salmon with Rice

INGREDIENTS

6 skinless filets of salmon

12 cups carrots cut quartered and sliced ¼ inch thick diagonally.

1 cup rice pilaf, uncooked

1 ½ cup water

1 teaspoon salt

¼ teaspoon freshly ground black pepper

½ cup slivered almonds (optional)

1 tablespoon chopped fresh mint

2 tablespoons extra virgin olive oil

6 sliced lemon wedges

DIRECTIONS

Preheat oven to 400 F. In a large baking dish, mix carrots rice and all the ingredients, slice the lemons and place in the refrigerator.

Place salmon fillets on top of rice mixture, season with salt and pepper. Cover dish with foil. Bake until the fish is no long pink, about 30-40 minutes.

Transfer to a platter, Fluff rice with fork. Serve with fish and slices of lemon on the side.

Makes 6 servings.

<Buon Appetito. Emilia>

RISOTTO CON FUNGHI ASSORTITE
Risotto with Mushrooms

INGREDIENTS

1pound shitake mushrooms

1 pound baby portabello mushrooms

2 tablespoons extra virgin olive oil

1 tablespoon margarine

½ teaspoon salt

¼ teaspoon freshly ground black pepper

½ cup minced shallot

12 oz. Arborio rice

1 cup white wine

4 cups water

½ cup grated Parmesan cheese

DIRECTIONS

In large nonstick pan heat oil and sauté shallots until tender, stirring occasionally, until golden and golden. Add mix mushrooms to the pan and cook until tender, about 5 minutes. Season with salt and pepper.

Meanwhile, heat margarine and sauté rice. Add wine and water, pinch salt and black pepper. Cover and cook at low medium heat for 10 minutes, or until all liquid is absorbed.

Mix in the rice mushrooms and half the cheese. Transfer into a serving platter. Garnish with remain cheese. Serve hot.

Makes 6-8 servings

<From my kitchen to your table. Enjoy Emi

PASTA & SAUCE
SALSA ALLA MARINARA
Basic Marinara Sauce

INGREDIENTS

1 28 oz can of tomato puree

1 28 oz can of crushed tomatoes

2 cloves of garlic, peeled and minced

½ cup onion, diced small

3 tablespoons extra virgin olive oil

4 basil leaves, chopped

1/2 teaspoon dried oregano flakes

2 tablespoons red wine

1 teaspoon salt

¼ teaspoon freshly ground black pepper

DIRECTIONS

In a saucepan, heat oil and sauté garlic and onion until golden and tender. Add tomatoes, basil leaves, salt, pepper, oregano and wine.

Cook for 30 minutes, if the sauce looks too thick add ½ cup water and cook for 30 minutes longer. Sauce need to be thick enough to stick to spaghetti or any pasta.

Test for seasoning before add the sauce to the pasta. Sauce can be kept in the refrigerator or frozen for 4-6 days.

<Happy cooking. Emilia>

EMILIA SALSA PICCANTE DI CALABRIA
Emilia Spice Tomato Sauce Calabrian Style

INGREDIENTS

2 bracioles (see recipe in the book)

6 country style spare ribs

6 meatballs (see recipe in the book)

6 hot Italian sausages

1 small cans tomatoes paste

1 28 oz can of crushed tomatoes

1 28 oz can of tomato puree

2 tablespoons olive oil

6 cloves of garlic, peeled and crushed

½ cup onion, minced

½ teaspoon crushed hot pepper

4 fresh basil leaves, (If fresh basil is not in season, use ½ teaspoon dry)

½ teaspoon oregano flakes

½ cup red wine (optional)

1 teaspoon salt

¼ teaspoon fresh ground red pepper

¼ cup vegetable oil

DIRECTIONS

In a large saucepan heat oil: sauté garlic and onions until golden or tender. Add tomatoes and all remaining ingredients, except for the vegetable oil. In a fry pan add vegetable oil and fry the meat until brown.

Partially cover the pan and cook slowly for 30 minutes. Add meatballs to the sauce and cook for 40 minutes longer. Taste for seasoning before adding to any pasta.

<Form my family to yours. Enjoy Emilia>

SALSA CON CARNE MACINATA
Meats Sauces

INGREDIENTS

¼ pound ground lean pork

¼ pound ground turkey

¼ pound ground beef

2 28 oz cans of peeled tomatoes

4 cloves of garlic, peeled and chopped

4 basil leaves, chopped

2 bay leaves

½ teaspoon dried oregano flakes

2 tablespoons extra virgin olive oil

1 cup red wine (optional)

1 teaspoon salt

½ teaspoon freshly ground black pepper

DIRECTIONS

In a large saucepan, heat oil and sauté garlic until golden. Add ground meats and sauté meats until browned. Add tomatoes and cook on low medium heat for 30 minutes.

Add all the remaining ingredients and cook for 30 minutes longer. Taste for seasoning before adding to spaghetti or any pasta or topping a pizza.

<Happy cooking. Emilia>

SALSA AL PESTO
Pesto Sauce

INGREDIENTS

4 cups fresh basil leaves

6 cloves of garlic, peeled

1 ½ cup extra virgin olive oil

½ teaspoon salt

½ teaspoon *freshly ground black pepper*

2 cups fresh Italian parsley

1 cup pine nuts

DIRECTIONS

In a food processor, place the basil leaves, parsley, pine nuts, garlic, salt and pepper. Cover and process until finely chopped. Add oil little at a time and process for 5 minutes or until mixture is pureed.

Pesto can be frozen, for whenever you need it, up to 5-6 months: or can be refrigerated up to 3-4 weeks. Serve over your favorite pasta.

Tips: If you have a small garden, take advantage of it. Plant basil and use it to make your marinara and pesto sauces

<Have fun. Emilia>

SALSA AL LIMONE E AGLIO PICCANTE
Spicy Garlic & Lemon Sauce

INGREDIENTS

4 cloves garlic, peeled and minced

3 tablespoons Italian seasoned breadcrumbs

1 tablespoon hot chili pepper flakes

2 tablespoons Italian parsley, chopped

¼ teaspoon freshly ground black pepper

½ teaspoon salt

3 tablespoons fresh lemon juice

½ cup dry white wine

DIRECTIONS

In a small bowl mix dry ingredients, then add wine and lemon juice 1 tablespoon each time. Stir to mix well after adding each tablespoon. This sauce should come out creamy.

When finished, adding the more wine if mixture is too dry, or add dry ingredients if mixture is too wet.

Spread over your favorite steak or fish dish. This can be made days before you need it. Put sauce into a plastic container and freeze until you need to use it.

<Have fun. Emilia>

SALSA ALLA GORGONZOLA
Blue Cheese Sauce

INGREDIENTS

8 oz Gorgonzola cheese

½ cup light cream

1 teaspoon fresh sage, finely chopped

6 sage leaves, shredded for garnish

¼ teaspoon salt

¼ teaspoon *freshly ground black pepper*

DIRECTIONS

In small saucepan heat Gorgonzola, cream, salt and ground black pepper heat until cream is hot and cheese is melted.

Add salt and black pepper and chopped sage. Toss sauce with your favor pasta or gnocchi.

This dish is very simple. Do not add cheese or other spices. Makes to add over 12 oz pasta or gnocchi.

<Enjoy Emilia>

FETTUCCINI ALFREDO

INGREDIENTS

1 pound fettuccini pasta

1 cup heavy cream

1 tablespoon margarine

½ teaspoon *freshly ground black pepper*

½ teaspoon salt

1 tablespoon fresh Italian parsley chopped

½ cup grated Parmesan cheese

DIRECTIONS

Cook pasta according to package directions, drain *al dente*. Meanwhile, in a large saucepan, melt margarine, add cream and bring to a boil. Reduce heat and simmer for 5 minutes, then add half the Parmesan cheese, pepper and pinch salt to taste.

Add fettuccine to the saucepan and toss well to combine ingredients and heat throughout, and season to taste.

Transfer fettuccine to a serving platter. Sprinkle with the remaining cheese and 1 tablespoon chopped parsley. Serve hot.

Makes 6 servings.

<Buon Appetito. Emilia>

EMILIA LINGUINIE PASTA CON PORKETTA AGIO E OILO
Emilia Linguini with Italia Pancetta, Garlic & Oil

INGREDIENTS

1 pound linguini pasta

6 oz dry Italian pancetta

4 cloves of garlic, peeled and chopped

2 tablespoons extra virgin olive oil

1 teaspoon oregano flakes

2 tablespoons fresh basil leaves, chopped

DIRECTIONS

In a small bowl, mix oil and garlic to blend well. Then heat garlic and oil and sauté until garlic is golden. Add pancetta and oregano to the pan, sauté for 2 minutes and set aside.

Cook linguine pasta according to package directions, drain, draining *al dente* and toss with pancetta mixture. Serve on a platter topped with chopped fresh basil.

Makes 6 servings.

<From my mother to me: and now to you. Emilia>

SPAGHETTI AL TONNO
Tuna & Spaghetti

1 pound thin spaghetti

2 14 oz cans of chunk tuna packed in water

2 tablespoons extra virgin olive oil

4 cloves garlic, peeled and chopped

1 15 oz can of peeled tomatoes

½ cup Italian parsley, chopped

½ teaspoon salt

½ teaspoon freshly ground black pepper

4 fresh basil leaves chopped

DIRECTIONS

In a skillet, sauté garlic until golden, then add tomatoes and crush with a fork. Add salt, pepper and basil leaves. Let cook tomatoes for 20 minutes on low medium heat. Add ¼ cup water and let cook for 5 minutes longer.

Rinse and drain tuna and add to the sauce. Cook for 5 minutes: or until sauce has a rich and thick consistency.

Cook spaghetti in a lightly salted boiling water according to package directions, drain *al dente* and pour into a serving bowl. Add tuna sauce mixture and toss gently.

Garnish with chopped parsley and serve hot.

Makes 6 servings.

<From me to you. Buon Appetito Emilia>

FARFALLE PASTA CON CARNE DI MANZO
Beef and Bows Alfredo

INGREDIENTS

1 pound beef, sirloin or top blade steak

½ cup chopped red bell pepper

8 oz sliced fresh mushrooms

1 pound bow tie pasta, freshly cooked *al dente*

2 package frozen asparagus, trimmed and cooked *al dente*

2 10 oz bottles of prepared light Alfredo sauce

¼ cup light toasted almonds

½ cup grated Parmesan cheese

½ teaspoon *freshly ground black pepper*

¼ teaspoon salt

Nonstick Pam spray

DIRECTIONS

Spray large skillet and sauté steak over medium-high heath about 3-5 minutes per each side or to desired doneness. For medium transfer steak to a cutting board when a meat thermometer registers 150F. and let it rest 10 minutes. Cut across the grain into thin slices.

Add peppers and mushrooms to hot skillet and sauté 3-5 minutes or until tender. Add sliced beef, pasta, asparagus, Alfredo sauce, and almonds, if desired. Heat for 2-3 minutes until hot throughout, stirring constantly, but do not boil. Top with cheese and pepper, if desired.

Makes 6 servings.

<Enjoy your meal. Emilia>

LINGUINI PASTA CON PESCE AL SUGO DI LIMONE
Lemon Seafood Linguini Pasta

INGREDIENTS

1 pound scallops

2 pounds mussels

1 pound medium shrimps

1 ½ cup extra dry white wine

12 tablespoons lemon zest

2 tablespoons extra virgin olive oil

1 tablespoon margarine

6 cloves garlic, peeled and sliced

1 cup red onion, chopped

1 pound or 1 bunch baby asparagus

1 pound linguini pasta

2 tablespoons fresh squeezed lemon juice

1 tablespoon fresh oregano chopped

¼ cup chopped Italian parsley

DIRECTIONS

Wash and trim asparagus and cut tender parts 1 inch long.

Scrub mussels and remove beards, peel shrimps and de-vein. Combine mussels with 1 cup wine in a sauce pan. Cover, bring to a boil and simmer until mussels are open.

Strain mussels and drain the liquid, reserving the liquid. Add the lemon zest to the liquid and simmer for 5 minutes. Cook linguini pasta in large pan with boil water and light salt, according to package directions and drain *al dente*.

In a large saucepan, heat oil and margarine, then sauté garlic and onion until golden. Add scallops, oregano, black pepper, salt, lemon juice, remaining wine and 2 cups of reserved liquid.

Simmer for 5 minutes. Add shrimps and mussels and cook for 4 minutes. Add cook linguini to the saucepan and toss well.

Transfer linguini to a large serving platter and garnish with chopped parsley. Serve hot. My hometown is near the ocean. Fish are sold very fresh every morning.

(Option: Toss ½ cup grated Parmesan cheese.)

Makes 6 servings.

<From my hometown to your table. Enjoy Emilia>

EMILIA PASTA PRIMAVERA
Emilia Spring Penne Pasta

DIRECTIONS

1 pound penne pasta

2 tablespoons extra virgin olive oil

4 cloves garlic, peeled and chopped

1 cup fresh tomatoes peeled, seeded and chopped

2 tablespoons fresh basil leaves chopped

1 cup zucchini, cut into 1-inch pieces

1 small red bell pepper, seeded and cut 1 inch pieces

1 small yellow bell pepper, seeded and cut 1 inch pieces

½ cup broccoli florets

1 cup button mushrooms, sliced

¼ cup celery chopped

1 teaspoon salt

½ teaspoon *freshly ground black pepper*

½ cup grated Parmesan cheese.

DIRECTIONS

In a large skillet, sauté garlic until golden. Add tomatoes and sauté for 2 minutes, and then add all the vegetables and ingredients. Reserve Parmesan cheese and ½ teaspoon salt for the pasta water. Simmer for 5-6 minutes.

Meanwhile cook pasta in a pan with boiling, lightly salt water according to package directions, drain *al dente*. Add penne pasta to skillet and toss with vegetables mixture. Transfer penne mixture into a serving platter. Sprinkle over the Parmesan cheese. Serve hot.

<Enjoy this light dish: is very health for you. Emilia>
MAIN COURSE MEALS

INVOLTINI DI TONNO
Fillet of Tuna roll up

INGREDIENTS

12 large tuna fillets

¼ cup extra virgin olive oil

½ cup yellow onion, minced

5 cloves garlic, chopped

1 pound tomatoes, peeled, seeded and chopped

1 sliced Italian bread, firm and crumbled

¼ cup skim milk

1 hard-boiled egg

1 egg beaten

¼ cup chopped Italian parsley

¼ teaspoon *freshly ground black pepper*

½ teaspoon salt

¼ cup grated Roman cheese

1 lemon sliced

DIRECTIONS

In large skillet heat oil, add onion and cook until tender, add garlic and sauté until golden. Add tomatoes, salt and black pepper. Cook for 20 minutes on low heat.

Soak bread into milk for 5 minutes and squeeze with your hand to dry out the bread and make into bread crumble.

Wash and dry filets, cut 2 filets fish into 1 inch-pieces. In a bowl, add bread, fish and remaining ingredients. Leave out the chopped parsley for garnish and mix well.

On a large wood surface, lay the filets out flat and spoon the mixture over them evenly. Roll up filets and secure with a toothpick: add the fish to the tomato sauce.

Cover and cook for 10 minutes on low medium heat. Transfer fish onto a serving platter, spoon the sauce over the roll up fish and serve hot.

This sauce is very tasty. To make a side of linguini pasta, double the tomatoes. You can cook 1 pound linguini and cook according the package directions. Serve hot

Makes 6 servings

<From my kitchen to your table. Buon Appetito. Emilia>

FILETTE DI PESCE E VEGETALI
　Fish filets Top with Vegetables

INGREDIENTS

6 large fish fillets, ½ inch thick

2 cups Roma tomatoes

½ cup sliced pitted black and green olives

1 tablespoon fresh oregano chopped

6 cloves garlic, peeled and chopped

½ teaspoon salt

½ teaspoon *freshly ground black pepper*

2 tablespoons Italian parsley chopped

½ cup red onion, sliced

3 cups assorted vegetables, broccoli spears, carrots and cucumbers

3 tablespoons pine nuts

DIRECTIONS

Preheat grill to medium. In a medium-sized bowl toss together tomatoes, olives, garlic, salt and black pepper. Rinse fish, and pat dry with paper towels. Tear off 6 18x12-inch pieces of heavy duty foil. Place 1 piece of fish in the center of each piece of foil. Top each fillets with some tomato mixture.

Bring up 2 opposite sides of foil and seal with a double fold. Fold remaining ends so the fish is completely enclosed, leaving some space for steam to expand. Grill foils packets for 4 minutes or until fish flakes easily when tested with a fork. (145 F.)

Open foil pockets. Transfer fish to a serving platter. Sprinkle with toasted pine nuts and vegetable mixture over the top. Serve hot.

Makes 6 servings.

<Enjoy Emilia>

SALSICCIE ITALIANE CON PEPERONI
Italian Sauce with fried Pepper

INGREDIENTS

6 Italian sausages

4 large bell peppers, red, green, yellow and orange

¾ cup red onion, large slices

¼ tablespoon red wine

½ cup tomatoes, peeled

½ teaspoon dried oregano

2 ¼ cups extra virgin olive oil

½ teaspoon salt

¼ *freshly ground black pepper*

DIRECTIONS

In a large oven skillet sauté onions and peppers until tender. Add sausage and cook for 5 minutes on low medium heat. Add the peeled tomatoes peel and remaining spices. Cook for 5 minutes.

Add wine and bring to a boil. Cover and transfer skillet to a preheat oven at 375 F. for 12-14 minutes. Serve hot with fresh Italian bread.

Makes 6 servings.

<Have fun in your kitchen. Emilia>

CARNE DI MAIALE ALLA GRIGLIA
  Grilled Pork Meats

INGREDIENTS

2 pork tenderloins about 2 pounds

1 tablespoon fresh oregano, chopped

1 large red onion, cut in half

2 bay leaves

2 chili peppers (optional)

4 cloves garlic, peeled and chopped

½ teaspoon sugar

1 cup red wine

¼ cup red or white vinegar

2 tablespoon soil?

1 teaspoon salt

1 teaspoon *freshly ground black pepper*

DIRECTIONS

Heat a charcoal grill until moderately hot. Meanwhile, combine all the ingredients except half the salt and black pepper in a saucepan with and add 1 cup water. Bring to boil and turn heat off.

With a slotted spoon transfer all vegetables into a serving platter. Sprinkle pork with salt and black pepper, and brown on each side until nearly cooked through (150 F), about 10-12 minutes.

Remove from remove from heat and let cool a 5 minutes and place in the marinade. If time allows, it is best to marinate for 2 hours or overnight in refrigerator.

Slice ¾ inch thick and serve at room temperature. Spoon marinated vegetables over each slice. For a quick service, marinate at least 3o minutes, then cut pork and serve.

With these methods: you can grill 8 pieces of pork chops then sliced pork chops individually and serve. This best served with bake beans or an Italian potato salad.

Makes 8 servings.

<Enjoy Emilia>

CONIGLIO ALLA CALABRESE
Rabbit Calabrian Style

INGREDIENTS

1 rabbit cut in small in pieces

2 tablespoons olive oil

2 bay leaves

2 fresh salvia leaves

2 cloves garlic, peeled and chopped

½ teaspoon salt

¼ teaspoon *freshly ground black pepper*

¼ cup dry white wine

2 tablespoons capers packed in oil

DIRECTIONS

Use fresh herbs if you can. Wash rabbit and dry with a paper towel. In a skillet, sauté rabbit until all the moisture disappears, about 4 minutes. Add oil garlic, bay leaves sage and salt and pepper.

Sauté rabbit over medium heat uncover until browned. Add wine and cook for 30 minutes. If wine is drying up, add little more or ½ cup water because the rabbit needs to be well done.

When rabbit is done, add cappers and serve next to baked potatoes and green salad.

Makess 6 servings.

<From my Regions to your tables enjoy. Emilia>

POLPA DI MAIALE AI CONTADINI
Lean Pork Meats Farm Style

INGREDIENTS

3 pond lean pork meats, cut into 1½ inch cubes

2 tablespoons breadcrumbs

2 tablespoons breadcrumbs

Few thin slices of Pecorino cheese

2 tablespoons olive oil

¼ cup Italian pancetta cut in small cubes

½ teaspoon salt

4 cloves garlic, peeled and chopped

½ teaspoon *freshly ground black pepper*

1 chili pepper chopped

½ cup red wine

2 bay leaves

½ teaspoon rosemary flakes

DIRECTIONS

In a large baking skillet add rabbit, pancetta, oil, garlic, salt and pepper. Sauté until browned. Add wine, rosemary and bay leaves. Cook on low medium heat for 5 minutes and add the white wine.

Cook uncovered for 5 minutes or until meat is no long pink. Cover top with breadcrumbs and grated cheese. Top with sliced Pecorino cheese. Bake in a preheated oven at 375 F. for 5 minutes or until top is browned. Serve with a side of brown rice.

Makes 6 servings.

<Buon Appetito. Emilia>

ARROSTO DI MAIALE PICCANTE
Spiced Grilled Steaks

DIRECTIONS

6 rib-eye steaks

1 ½ tablespoons kosher salt

½ tablespoon ground cumin

1 tablespoon *freshly ground black pepper*

1 tablespoon cayenne pepper

DIRRECTIONS

Heat grill for cooking. In a small bow, stir together all spice. With your hand, rub spice mixture equally over the steaks both sides, pressing well for the spices to stick to steaks.

Brush grill with oil: grill for 4 minutes on each side. You can insert thermometer horizontally into thickest parts. For medium rare, cook until 140F. For well done, cook until 150F.

Transfer steaks to a serving platter. Serve with a green salad.

Makes 6 servings.

<Buon Appetito. Emilia>

TORTELLINI E PROSCIUTTO

INGREDIENTS

6 oz prosciutto Parma, sliced 1/8 thick

2 pound fresh cheese tortellini

1 cup frozen sweet peas

1 tablespoon margarine

2 tablespoon extra virgin olive oil

2 tablespoons flour

2 cups heavy cream

¼ cup grated Parmesan cheese

Pinch fresh black pepper

DIRECTIONS

Defrost the peas and set aside. Cook tortellini according to package directions. Drain tortellini, cover and put aside.

In large skillet, melt margarine, add flour and stir constantly with a whisk until thoroughly blended. Add heavy cream and bring to a light boil, until the cream mixture becomes yellow in color.

Add prosciutto and sweet peas to cream mixture and return to heat. Butter a large baking dish, spread tortellini in and cover with cream mixture. Sprinkle with Parmesan cheese and lay sliced prosciutto on top. Bake uncover, in a preheated oven, at 375F. for 15 minutes or until top is light golden brown.

Makes 8 servings.

<Enjoy Emilia>

FILETTO DI VITELLA AL COGNAC
Veal Chops with Cognac Sauce

INGREDIENTS

6 center cut veal chops, 1 ¼ thick: fat removed

¼ cup cognac

1 tablespoon margarine

4 cups sliced mixed mushrooms, shiitake and cremini

4 cloves garlic, peeled and chopped

½ tablespoon rosemary leaves chopped

1 tablespoon Italian parsley chopped

1 minced shallot

6 fresh sage leaves for decorations

1 tablespoon olive oil

½ cup heave cream

1 teaspoon salt

½ teaspoon *freshly ground black pepper*

DIRECTIONS

Sprinkle the chops with salt and pepper. In large skillet, heat margarine over low medium heat. Sauté veal chops, cover and cook until brown: about 4 minutes.

Transfer chops on serving platter, cover to stay warm. In the same skillet, add 1 tablespoon oil and sauté garlic until golden. Add shallot and sauté for 30 seconds; shallots need very little time to cook.

Add mushrooms, parsley, salt and pepper, cook for 30 second: add cognac and cook for 1 minute. Add cream and simmer on low medium heat for 1 minute.

Pour the mixture over the chops. Garnish each chops with sage. Serve hot.

Makes 6 servings.

<Enjoy Emilia>

PETTO DI POLLO ARROSTO CON VEGETALE
Grilled Chicken & Vegetables

INGREDIENTS

6 skinless boneless chicken breast, halved

2 tablespoon extra virgin olive oil

1 medium onion, cut in thin wedges

2 medium bell peppers, green and red, cut into ¼-inch wide strips

1 large Italian zucchini, cut in 2 ½ sticks

½ teaspoon salt

1 teaspoon lemon pepper mix

DIRECTIONS

Mix 1 tablespoon oil and lemon pepper in a Ziploc bag. Add chicken and shake to coat. Heat a stovetop grill pan over medium heat. Transfer chicken into the hot grill, heat a broil to medium heat.

Broil chicken 4 minutes each side until chicken is cooked through. Remove to a cutting board and let it stand for 5 minutes. Meanwhile heat remaining oil in a large non stick pan. Over medium heat add onion, red and green peppers and sauté for 3 minutes until crisp.

Add zucchini, sauté vegetables 3 minutes long and season with salt. Sliced the chicken and serve with lemon wedges and vegetables.

Makes 4 servings.

<From my kitchen to your table. Enjoy Emilia>

CONGHIGLIE RIPIENE AL SALMONE E RICOTTA
Pasta shells Staffed with Salmon & cheese

INGREDIENTS

1pound pasta shells, about 16 shells

1 tablespoon extra virgin olive oil

1 clove garlic peeled and chopped

1 cup tomatoes peeled, seeded and chopped

1 pound ricotta cheese

3 oz. smoked salmon

1 egg separated (white from yolk)

2 fresh basil leaves

½ teaspoon salt

½ teaspoon *freshly ground black pepper*

DIRECTIONS

Preheat oven to 400 F.

Cook pasta shells in light salt boil water according to package directions. Drain and set aside.

In a small skillet, heat oil and sauté garlic until golden. Add tomatoes, a pinch of salt and black pepper. Cook for 5 minutes and set aside.

In a blender, mix the ricotta cheese and salmon, and egg yolk. Blend until it makes a soft and creamy filling. Transfer mixture into a bowl. Whisk the egg white until fluffy and at soft peak stage and fold into the mixture.

Stuff the shells with the ricotta mixture: Grease a baking pan with vegetable oil spray, and put the shells into baking pan. Cover with tomato sauce and bake for 15 to 20 minutes. Serve hot.

Makes 4 servings.

<Buon Appetito. Emilia>

ERBE MISTE PER CARNI
Mix Herbs for Meats

2 tablespoons parsley flakes

1 tablespoon lemon zest

2 tablespoons thyme

2 tablespoons chopped fresh rosemary or 1 tablespoon of rosemary flakes

1 tablespoon garlic powder

1 tablespoon salt

1 tablespoon ground black pepper.

DIRECTIONS

In a small bowl, mix all the ingredients. Sprinkle over poultry during cooking or use in a shaker at the table.

Store any extra spice in a tightly covered glass container in the refrigerator.

You can make this a day ahead to save time.

<Have fun. Emilia>

ARROSTO DI VITELLA AL LIMONE
Lemon Veal Roast

2 pounds of boneless veal roasts

3 tablespoons olive oil

2 tablespoons white vinegar

2 tablespoons cool water

1 teaspoon salt

2 tablespoons sage chopped

2 cloves garlic, chopped

2 tablespoons flour

DIRECTIONS

In a small contain, mix oil, vinegar, water, lemon pepper, salt and garlic. Rub mixture over the veal roast. Preheat oven at 350 F. place roast fat side down, on rack shallow roasting pan. Pour remaining dressing over the roast.

Cook roast for 45 minutes, then insert meat thermometer into thickest part of roast. The meat thermometer should register at 150 F.

Let the roast stand for 10 minutes before cutting. Veal takes less time to cook then pork or beef.

Bring the roasting pan over to the stove burners. Add ½ cup water and flour, stirring over low heat until the pan juices thicken. Slice roast into pieces ½ inch thick and transfer to a serving platter. Pour over the roast the gravy from the baking pan and serve with a potato or green salad.

Makes 6 servings.

<Enjoy Emilia.>

FILETTI DI MAIALE RIPIENI
Staffed Pork Chops

INGREDIENTS

6 large pork chops, cut 1 inch thick

3 tablespoons flavored Italian breadcrumbs

1 tablespoon fresh sage finely chopped

6 tablespoon shredded Fontina cheese

6 slices Fontina cheese

½ teaspoon *freshly ground black pepper*

1 teaspoon salt

2 tablespoons Italian parsley chopped

4 cloves garlic peeled and chopped

Pam spray

Fresh rosemary springs for garnish

DIRECTIONS

Make a deep pocket, with your knife, into each pork chop. In a small bowl mix all the ingredients, leaving out the salt and pepper. Divided the stuffing into 6 portions and put inside the pork chops. Secure chops pockets with wooden toothpicks. Preheat oven at 400 F. Rub pork chops with salt and pepper.

Grease a baking pan with Pam spray. Lay pork chops into the pan and bake for 30 minuets, or until the juices run clear. Add the slice Fontina cheese over chops and bake for additional 2 minutes. Serve with a side dish of brown rice and garnish with sprigs rosemary leaves.

Makes 6 servings.

<From my kitchen to your table. Enjoy Emilia.>

SALMONE E POMODORI ARROSTITE
Salmon Fillets with Roast Tomatoes

INGREDIENTS

6 large tomatoes cut in half

2 tablespoons extra virgin olive oil

6 piece salmon fillets, about 3 oz each

¾ pound sliced mushrooms, your choice

1 pound green beans, trimmed

¼ cup grated Parmesan cheese

6 lemon wedges

DIRECTIONS

In a large roasting pan drizzle tomatoes with olive oil. Preheat the oven to 425 F and cook the roast for 30 minutes. Add the salmon and mushrooms for the final 10 minutes of cooking time.

Meanwhile cook green beans in boiling salt water for 5 minutes or until just cooked, drain well. Transfer fish and tomatoes mixture onto a serving plate, and add a side of green beans.

Sprinkle Parmesan cheese over fish mixture and garnish with a lemon wedge.

<Buon Appetito. Emilia>

DESERTS

VARIAZIONE PER DECORARE LE TORTE
Toppings Variations for Cake

INGREDIENTS

1 cup powdered sugar

2 tablespoons water

2 tablespoon lemon extract

1 tablespoon lemon juice (optional)

DIRECTIONS

In a bowl mix all 3 ingredients until softened and creamed. Spread over the cake with wood spatula.

INGREDIENTS

8 oz cream cheese softened

1 pound powdered sugar

1 stick softened butter

½ cups sliced almonds for topping

The same direction as above. Decorated frosting with sliced almonds.

INGREDIENTS

1 cup confections sugar

¼ cup heavy cream

1 tablespoon butter

1 tablespoon coffee brandy

DIRECTIONS

Mix all ingredients with an electric mixer until stiff and smooth.

Use for filling the cake or to decorate the top of the cake.

CLASSICA TORTA AL CIOCCOLATO
Classic Chocolate Cake

INGREDIENTS

1 cup butter softened

½ cup vegetables shortening

2 ¼ cups granulated sugar

5 large eggs

3 cups cake flour, sifted

½ teaspoon baking powder

¾ cup evaporate milk

¼ cup water

2 teaspoons vanilla extract

ICING

8 oz cream cheese softened

¼ cup butter softened

4 cups confectioners sugar

1 teaspoon vanilla extract

DIRECTIONS

Preheat oven to 350 F. Arrange racks to the center of the oven. Grease and dust with flour, 3 round layer spring form cake pans. Line bottoms with rounds of waxed paper.

Cream butter and shortening with sugar until very light and fluffy. Add eggs one at time, beating well after each egg. Sift flour with baking pour, set aside.

Combine milk, water and vanilla extract. Add flour mixture to batter alternating with milk mixture, begin and ending with flour.

Divide batter evenly among pans and bake 30-40 minutes or until toothpick inserted in the center comes out clean. Cool cakes in the pans for 10 minutes, then turn out onto racks to complete cooling.

ICING

DIRECTIONS

Beat cream cheese with butter until smooth. On medium speed, gradually beat with confectioners sugar until light and fluffy. Blend in cocoa and vanilla extract: continue beating until frosting is smooth.

Spread generously and smooth between layers and cover the sides and top of cake.

<Indulge your self with a thin slice. Emilia>

TORTA AL CIOCCOLATO FACILE
Easy One Bowl Chocolate Cake

INGREDIENTS

1 cup all purpose flour

1cup sugar

½ cup unsweetened cocoa powder

½ teaspoon baking soda

¼ teaspoon baking powder

¼ teaspoon salt

¾ cup milk

1/3 cup cooking olive oil, extra virgin

¾ cup milk

1 teaspoon vanilla

1 egg

Powdered sugar for dust

DIRECTIONS

Preheat oven to 350 F. Grease and lightly flour a 9-inch, round, spring-form baking pan. In a large bowl, mix combine flour, sugar, cocoa, powder, baking soda, baking powder and salt. Add milk, oil and vanilla. Beat with electric mixer on low speed until all ingredients combined, about 2 minutes.

Add egg and beat for two minutes longer. Pour batter into prepared pan. Bake for 35 minutes or until wood toothpick comes out clean. Cool cake thoroughly on wire rack. Before serving, sprinkle on the powdered sugar. Transfer onto a serving cake platter.

<Enjoy Emilia>

CROSTA DI FRAGOLE
Strawberry Pie

INGREDIENTS

Pastry

2 cups all-purpose flour

½ cup butter, softened

¼ cup confectioners' sugar

Filling

3 cups prepared pudding pie filling mix or custard

Topping

4 cups whole strawberries, hulled

½ cup red current jelly, melted

DIRECTIONS

Mix together, butter and confections sugar. Make dough into a ball, wrap in a plastic wrap, and chill for 30 minutes. Press dough into 9 inch rounds into a spring-form pan. Pick through with fork and chill for 30 minutes.

Bake in preheated oven at 400 F. for 8 minutes or until golden brown. Allow pastry to cool thoroughly; remove pastry from pan and place on serving plate. Spoon over the pudding and pie filling. Top with whole strawberries. Brush strawberries with melted jelly.

Chill pie until ready to serve.

<From my kitchen to your table. Enjoy Emilia>

PANNA COTTA
Italian Custard

INGREDIENTS

½ cup sugar

3 ½ teaspoons unflavored gelatin

3 cups buttermilk

1 cup fresh chopped fruit, whatever is in season

½ cups toasted pine nuts

DIRECTIONS

In a medium saucepan, combine sugar and gelatin and add cream. Heat and stir until gelatin is dissolved. Remove from heat and stir in the buttermilk.

Pour custard into 12 individual custard cups, cover and chili for 6 to 8 hours, or until set.

To serve, immerse bottom of the cups into hot water: run a clean knife around edge to loosen. Invert onto dessert plate. Serve with fresh fruit and toasted pine nuts.

<Have fun! Emilia>

TORTA ALLA MOCA
Mocha Cake

INGREDIENTS

4 eggs separated

½ cup water

½ cup sugar

2 tablespoons instant espresso coffee powder

4 tablespoons cocoa powder

1 cup all-purpose flour

2 tablespoons baking powder

FROSTING

1 cup confectioners sugar

¼ cup heavy cream

1 tablespoon butter

1 tablespoon coffee brandy

DIRECTIONS

With an electric mixer beat egg yolks and sugar. Add water and espresso coffee. Then add cocoa powder, flour and baking powder.

In a separate bowl beat egg whites until fluffy and stiff, and then fold into flour mixture with wood spatula.

Grease two, 8 inch, round, spring-form cake pans and add a round circle piece of wax paper onto bottom of the pan.

Bake for 20 minutes or until a toothpick comes out clean. Transfer cake to a rack to cool. Mix all frosting ingredients with an electric mixer until stiff and smooth.

Put one cake on a serving plate: spread frosting over the entire cake, top with second cake and cover entire cake with frosting.

Cover and refrigerate cake for 2 hours before serving.

<Have a thin slice. Emilia>

TORTA SEMPLICE
Easy Cake

INGREDIENTA

2 cups flour

7 eggs separated

1 cup sugar

3 tablespoons baking powder

4 oz vegetable oil

6 oz water

Pinch salt

DIRECTIONS

Preheat oven at 350 F.

Beat egg yolk and sugar until creamed. Add oil and water and beat well. Sift flour and baking pour and add to the eggs mixture.

Beat white eggs until soft peaks are formed. With a wood spatula, fold eggs whites into the cake mixture.

Grease a 9-inch, round, spring-form cake pan. Place into oven and bake for 90 minutes uncovered.

Serve with scoop of your favorite ice cream.

<Indulge your self with a thin slice. Emilia>

EMILIA BISCOTTI ALLE NOCCIOLINI
Emilia Hazelnuts Cookie

INGREDIETS

4 eggs

½ cup granulated sugar

16 oz honey

1 teaspoon cinnamon

2 teaspoons baking powder

2 tablespoon tangerine zest

5 cups Arthur King flour

½ cup olive oil

2 cups hazelnuts, roasted, peeled and chopped

DIRECTIONS

Preheat oven at 400 F.

With electric mixer, beat eggs and sugar for 2 minutes, then add honey and beat until mixture is combined. Add baking powder, cinnamon, oil and tangerine zest, mix everything is combined well.

Add flour 1 cup at a time and blend well, then add hazelnuts 1 cup at a time. Divide the dough into 4 portions. Sprinkle flour on a wood surface and roll each portion into 16 inches long by 2 inches thick.

Cover a large cookie baking pan with waxed paper, space the cookie log 4 inches apart and brush with beaten eggs or milk.

Bake for 20-25 minutes. Let the cookie cool down before cutting
Slice them half inch wide diagonally. If you prefer the biscotti to be extra crunchy, reduce oven temperatures to 300 F. and return them to the hot oven for 1 minute.

<From my kitchen to your table. Enjoy Emilia>

BISCOTTI PREFERITI DI PAP' CON IL VINO BIANCO
My Father's Special Cookies with White Wine

INGREDIENTS

3 cups flour

1 cups white wine

1 egg

¾ cups sugar

1 teaspoon fennel seed

1 pinch salt

DIRECTIONS

On a wood surface add flour and make a well in the center. Add all the ingredients and work with your hands until you have smooth dough.

Roll it out into long logs. Cut 5 inch long pieces and seal both ands together to make a small circle.

Dip the top part of each cookie into a dish of granulated sugar, and then arrange them on a lightly greased and floured baking pan with the sugar covered side facing up.

Bake in a preheated 375F oven for 20 minutes. Let cookies cool.

These cookies are well appreciated at parties with a glass of good wine.

<Enjoy! And have fun. Emilia>

MISCELLANEOUS

APPETIZERS
Appetizers

1 package frozen pastry shells

1 can 10 oz chicken soup

½ cup milk

2 tablespoons white wine

1 tablespoon dried parsley flakes

A dash of onion and garlic pour

1 teaspoon brown sugar

1/2 teaspoon onion powder

1 ¾ cups cooked ham

1 3/5 cup fresh, tender asparagus, cut in 1 inch pieces (cooked and pat dry, drain with paper towel)

¾ cup shredded Swiss cheese

DIRECTIONS

Bake pastry shells according to package directions.

Mix soup, milk, wine, parsley, sugar and onion in saucepan. Stir in asparagus, ham and cheese. Heat throughly.

Serve in a pastry shells. Makes 6 serving.

<Have fun. Emilia>

CROSTINI ALLA CANNELLA
Cinnamon Bread Sticks

INGREDIENTS

1 package dry yeast

1/3 cup warm water

1 cup warm, skim milk

3 eggs, beaten

½ cup sugar

½ cup margarine, melted

6 cups all-purpose flour

FILLING

2 egg whites

½ cup brown sugar

2 teaspoons cinnamon

DIRECTIONS

In a large bowl, dissolve yeast in warm water. Add milk, margarine, eggs, sugar and 4 cups of flour. Beat all ingredients until smooth. Stir in remaining flour and work until forms a soft dough. Turn dough over a lightly flour surface, knead until smooth and elastic (about 5 to 6 minutes).

Place dough in a greased bowl. Turn once to grease the top. Cover and let stand for 2 hours or until double the volume. Punch dough down and turn onto flour surface. Divide dough into 4 pieces. Roll each piece into a thin, square, flat dough, about ½ inch thick. Beat egg whites until soft peaks form. Brush eggs white over the dough, sprinkle over cinnamon and brown sugar.

Cut dough 2 ½ inches wide and 12 inches long. Roll all the dough pieces to make a round stick. Continue this method with the remainding dough and pinch seams to seal, and pinch ends to seal. Place each roll seam side down in a greased baking pan. Cover with a dish cloth and let rise in a warm place for 30 minutes. Bake at 350 F for 15 to 20 minutes or until golden or light brown.

Remove from pans to wire racks to cool. Serve hot or cold at your party. This can be kept in a plastic container with a cover for 1 week or frozen up to 1 month.

<Have your children or grandchildren help you out. This can be fun! Emilia>

PEPERONI ALLA CALABRESE
Calabrian Peppers

INGREDIENTS

4 large bell peppers, red, yellow, green and orange

2 tablespoons olive oil, extra virgin

½ cup grated Romaine cheese

1 cup Italian flavored breadcrumbs

3 Italian sausages, case removed

2 cooked eggs, peeled and chopped

1 tablespoon fresh chopped parsley

¼ teaspoon fresh ground black pepper

Vegetable oil for spray

DIRECTIONS

Wash and dry peppers, cut top, and remove seeds. In a small bowl add breadcrumbs, cheese, meat from sausage, chopped eggs, salt, black pepper, oil, and parsley.

Combine mixture and divide mixture into equal portions. Spoon mixture onto peppers. Preheat oven at 375 F. Spray a baking dish with vegetable oil. Bake and cover for 30 minutes, uncover and bake for additional 6 to 8 minutes or until top is golden brown.

Serve as side dish next to a green salad

<From the southern Italy to your tables, enjoy. Emilia>

PER ARROSTIRE L'AGLIO
How to Roast Garlic

Slice the top using a sharp knife. Drizzle top with oil. Wrap with aluminum foil and bake at 400 F for 30 minutes.

Squeeze garlic to remove the pulp once it cools. If you want to puree the garlic, place the garlic into a blender or food processor. This garlic can be spread over bruschetta or incorporated into risotto and a spaghetti dish.

To make garlic oil, add crushed garlic into a jar with 2 cups olive oil extra virgin. Seal with lid and refrigerate up to 1 month.

Roasted garlic can only be refrigerated up to 1 week.

<Have fun. Emilia>

LIQUID MEASURE VOLUME EQUIVALENTS

1 teaspoon	= less than 1/8 teaspoon
1 tablespoon	= 3 teaspoons
2 tablespoons	= 1 fluid ounces
4 tablespoons	= 1/4 cup
5 tablespoons	= 1/3 cup
8 tablespoons	= ½ cup
3/8 cup	= ¼ cup
5/8 cup	= ½ cup
1 cup	= 8 ounce
16 tablespoons	= 1 cup
1 gill	= ½ cup
1 pint	= 16 ounces
1 quart	= 4 cups
1 gallon	= 4 quarts

ABOUT THE AUTHOR

Emilia was born and raised in Calabria, Italy. She came to this country at age 26. Emilia married her husband, Peter, who is also from Italy, at the age of 28. Their first son, Alberto, was born in 1972. Married to his wife Kristine, they now have two beautiful daughters, Cara Mia, and Gianna Maria.

Their daughter Silvia was born in 1974 and is now married to her husband Shawn. They have a beautiful son named Anthony Michael.

As a young girl Emilia enjoyed cooking with her mother and now passed that same love to her family. Her recipes have been in her family for many years. Now she is sharing with you her own special taste of Southern Italy, Calabria.

She enjoys embroidery, sewing, knitting, reading and writing.

Her love from her family and God keeps her strong from her disease of asthma.

Her three beautiful grandchildren give Emilia strength and motivation to keep strong faith while living with asthma, and learn more each day what she can about this disease.

978-0-595-36854-9
0-595-36854-9

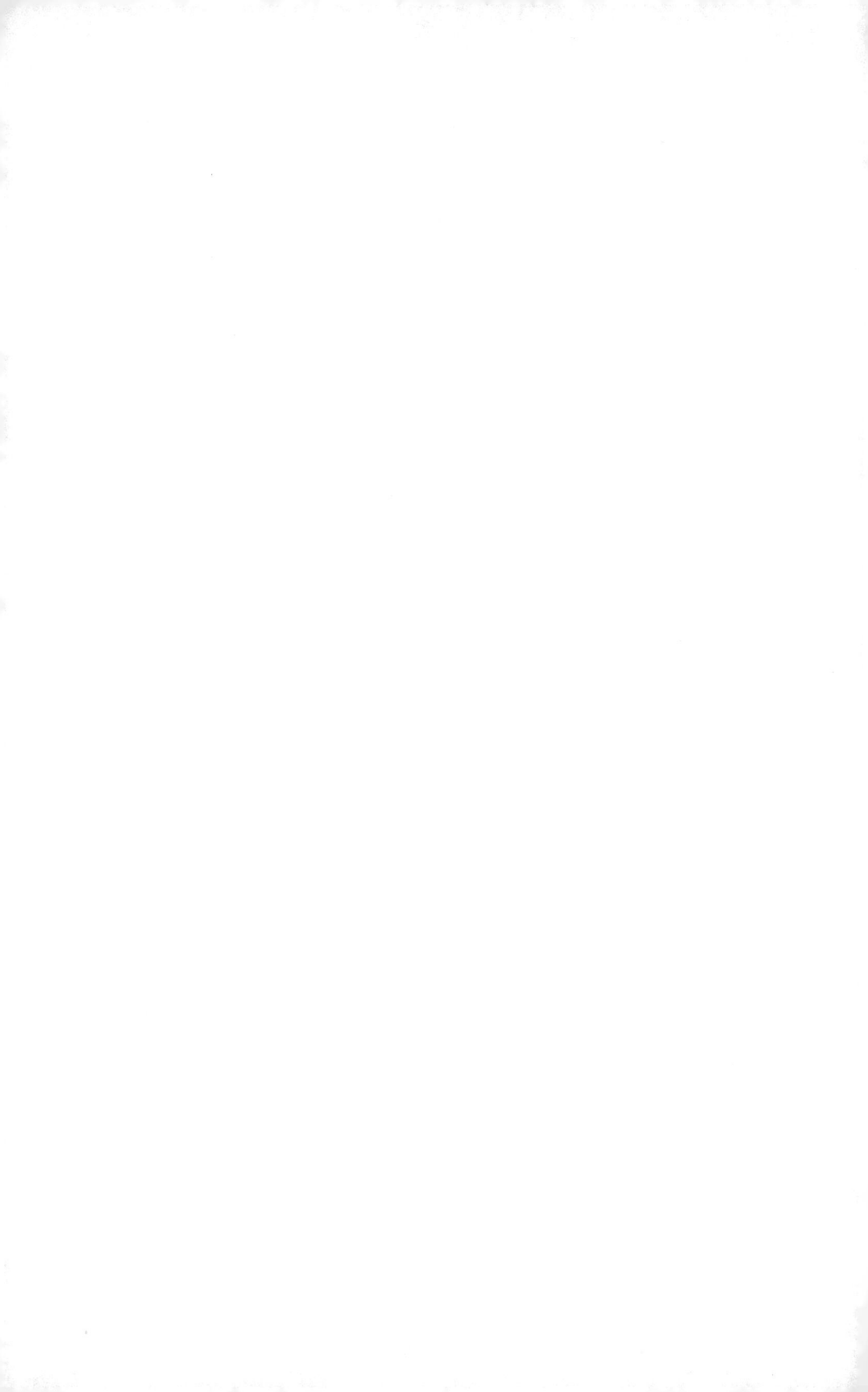

www.ingramcontent.com/pod-product-compliance
Lightning Source LLC
Chambersburg PA
CBHW030312290526
45785CB00001B/317